THE ULTIMATE MEMORY ACTIVITY BOOK

130 Puzzles and Recreational Ideas for
People Living with Memory Loss

Alexis Olson, PhD

PUZZLES BY **Phil Fraas**

**ROCKRIDGE
PRESS**

For general information on our other products and services or to obtain technical support, please contact our Customer Care Department within the United States at (866) 744-2665, or outside the United States at (510) 253-0500.

Rockridge Press publishes its books in a variety of electronic and print formats. Some content that appears in print may not be available in electronic books, and vice versa.

Interior and Cover Designer: Emma Hall
Art Producer: Hannah Dickerson
Editors: Lori Tenny and Samantha Holland
Production Editor: Emily Sheehan

All illustrations used under license from Shutterstock.com

Author photo courtesy of Jonathan Walker

ISBN: Print 978-1-64739-725-8
R0

To my teachers, patients, and loved ones
who shared their memories with me, which
helped me better understand my own.

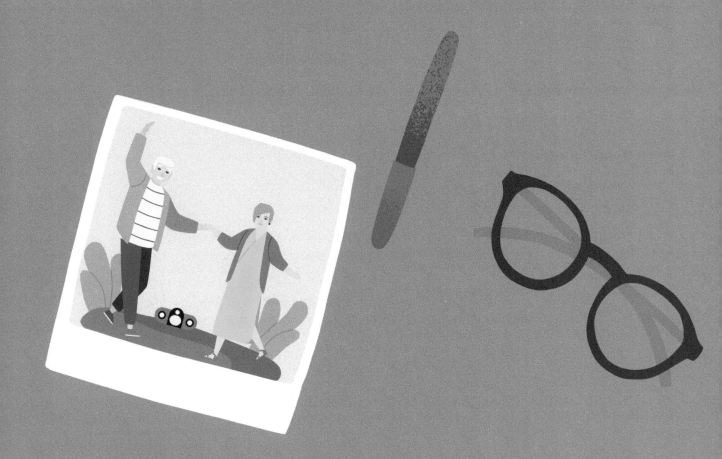

CONTENTS

CHAPTER 4:
Let's Do This! 30 Engaging Activity Tips 139

INTRODUCTION

Adapting to changes in our abilities can be a precarious task. Whether you are facing age-related changes, recovery from brain injury, or memory loss due to a neurological disorder like Alzheimer's disease or a vascular condition like a stroke, it can be a time of tremendous uncertainty. The road can be marked with frustration and surprise and require persistence and encouragement.

As a clinical neuropsychologist, I work with people and their loved ones as they encounter memory loss of varying degrees and origins. I assess how changes in thinking skills might affect mood or engagement in everyday activities, then provide guidance and interventions designed to optimize how my patients function in these areas.

Memory loss can certainly be a scary experience, so I try to make it more manageable. I work closely with people who are having difficulty with tasks that were once automatic, like remembering names or recent conversations. Together we navigate how to best integrate this new version of their abilities into a rewarding daily life. We practice new styles of learning information or training family members to give assistive cues. Sources of feedback and encouragement can take someone from giving up to giving it another go.

Throughout this book, I provide information on how to support brain health by facilitating good nutrition, effective physical and mental exercise, quality sleep, and other healthy practices, with the goal of maintaining memory and overall brain health. Research shows that taking a holistic approach to health helps us address the mechanisms that influence brain health and can potentially inhibit or slow the progression of memory loss.

Mental engagement is a key aspect of brain health that is richly represented throughout this book. I've included activities of varying levels of difficulty, and the puzzle author has designed word and number games to challenge and entertain you. If you find yourself getting discouraged, take a breather, and approach it again with fresh eyes. Have fun!

HOW TO USE THIS BOOK

Reading this book means that you're already accessing a tool to optimize brain health and cognitive functioning. I'll provide many engaging activities at a range of challenge levels, ranging from 1 to 3, with 1 being the easiest.

Chapters 2 and 3 are composed entirely of word and number puzzles of gradually increasing difficulty; some puzzles contain helpful hints. You'll find the solutions in the answer key at the back of the book. Chapter 2 is a compilation of crossword puzzles, word searches, and word scrambles of various themes that help orient you to some of the answers. Chapter 3 turns up your numeric game using Sudoku, number search, and number fill-in puzzles. Chapter 4 is composed of a variety of brain-stimulating activity ideas to try during your recreational time. These include exploring your surroundings with fresh eyes, expanding your creative skills through writing and music, making things with your hands, and other activities. Each activity targets a different type of cognitive ability (such as attention or prospective memory). Some activities require simple props, such as paper and a pen or basic gardening items, while others simply require you to have your mind turned to the "ready" position.

Keep in mind that there is no right way to move through this book. Given the wide range of activities and challenge levels, you can jump in at any point that works best for you. Feel free to skip around or proceed front to back. The only requirement is that you strike a balance between challenging yourself to the best of your abilities and also enjoying yourself. Some activities will likely feel more difficult than others, but persistence will help your brain stay as strong as it can be.

So, grab your pencil, and start filling in some of the 100 brain-stimulating puzzles in the next two chapters, or jump to the last chapter for some interesting and mentally engaging activity ideas if you're ready to get moving. Practicing the challenges that follow will help keep your mind engaged and your brain firing and wiring!

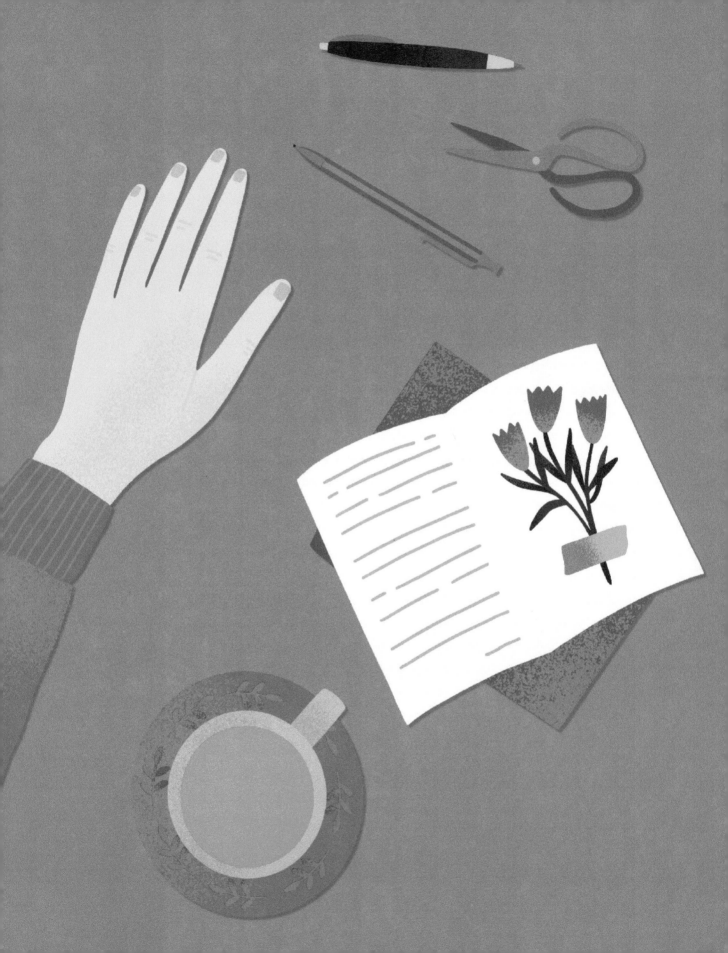

CHAPTER 1

Keeping Your Tool Sharp

Before I learned to drive, my mom said I needed to learn what was under the hood of a typical car. Though I could make it from here to there without much trouble, she knew that if I ever found myself on the side of the road, I'd want to know what to look for within this huge piece of machinery. We can think of our path through life in a similar way, without knowing all of the ins and outs of our mind. It sure is nice to have some insight into the mechanics of thinking, though—especially when we run into cognitive hiccups.

When we talk about memory, most people think of one subtype called long-term memory—our ability to recall past events and information. Unlike the common "file drawer" metaphor, where we neatly file each memory away and pull it out in its pristine state, our memories are actively and dynamically processed. They are reconstituted and colored by a combination of our past experiences, current environmental cues, and our current physical and emotional state. For this reason, whether one already experiences memory difficulties or not, the important task of tending to our physical brain and body, as well as our emotional needs, is highlighted across memory research and practice. In this chapter, you will be introduced to ways in which memory can be adversely affected, the components of optimizing brain health, and how to engage your mind to harness memory to the best of your abilities.

LIVING WITH MEMORY LOSS

Many conditions affect memory, including brain injury, neurodegenerative conditions like Alzheimer's disease, and significant mood difficulties. It's helpful to review the mechanisms that make memory function to understand why these can affect memory.

Memory begins with **attention**—our ability to hone in on the sensations that compose an experience. Let's say you're at the park and see a rabbit nearby. Your senses mark the rabbit's color and movement, the way the grass moves under its feet, and the flowers it nibbles. Your attention has to let go of or block out all surrounding activities—trees, children playing, a bus driving by—to focus on this rabbit. Your attention has been directed and held to the small scene in front of you involving this little animal.

Next comes **emotion and elaboration**. If you have no interest in rabbits, your attention will likely move quickly toward something of more interest to you, like the people playing touch football on the field. If you do like rabbits, you'll contemplate the fluffy animal you see and have the urge to pet it. As you watch it nibble flowers, you'll think of the sweet clover, as if you have enjoyed nibbling on it, which creates an emotional charge of rewarding enjoyment. This charge, sent from the emotion centers of your brain, facilitates holding this experience of the rabbit in your short-term memory. By elaborating—making associations with preexisting memories, like the clover—you establish even more grounds for remembering this event.

When you leave the park, you use your **short-term memory** to keep the experience of the rabbit alive. Your short-term memory functions as a sort of temporary holding tank. It must be accessed frequently, or the details will drift away in a matter of seconds. Reviewing this experience and describing to yourself or a friend all the details of observing that rabbit and the associations you made to it creates further impressions on your brain. Your brain then works to move these details from your short-term memory to your **long-term memory**, where they are stored for later access.

One might say a memory has formed during this long-term memory stage. One brain structure key to effective long-term memory is the hippocampi (hippocampus, singular)—two small, seahorse-shaped structures located on either side of the inner area of your brain. Sleep is very important at this stage. Studies suggest that the bulk of consolidation, or moving information from short- to long-term memory, occurs in deep slumber.

But why store that memory if you're not going to use it on the right occasion? Once information is in your long-term memory, the task of calling it up at just the right time and in as much detail as possible can be tricky. The process of recalling memories from our long-term memory takes many forms.

▶ **Declarative memory.** We often want to share experiences with others, which flexes our declarative memory, or our ability to state the details of our experience or knowledge. This occurs in two ways:

- **Episodic memory.** This is our ability to recall the details of a given event or episode. If someone asked us where and when we saw that rabbit, our episodic memory holds details like the location of the park, the time of day, what we did right before visiting the park, and who we were with. It can be troublesome to find that we don't recall the name of the park, despite visiting it multiple times each month.

- **Semantic memory.** In the case that we don't recall the name of the park, our episodic memory is affected by difficulties in semantic memory, the web of names and information built over our lifetime. This web of info can be independent of our personal experience. We don't have to have visited the park before to know where it is on a map or have owned a rabbit as a pet to know that they like carrots.

▶ **Procedural memory.** This more resilient type of memory results from repeatedly carrying out a series of steps. We can carry out these steps without necessarily being able to verbalize what they are. The action just happens. Procedural memory occurs during activities like riding a bike, fixing a favorite recipe, or doing a set of well-practiced dance moves. Procedural memory is often preserved in cases of memory impairment when declarative memory is compromised.

▶ **Prospective memory.** Prospective memory involves just that: your prospects. It considers the future—those tasks you need to do tomorrow (or was it the day after tomorrow?). What are the prospects of remembering to preheat the oven in time to eat dinner by 6:30 p.m. tomorrow? They're actually kind of low, so that's where timers and alerts come in handy. Cues can help with each of this type of memory.

As you can see, there are a variety of steps and details involved in each type of memory, each aligning with a different brain structure or process. And as stated earlier, the hippocampi, repetition, and sleep are all very useful in making new memories. People will experience memory loss in a variety of different ways, depending on which step in the memory-forming process or area of the brain is affected. In any case, one thing is true, however: Maintaining brain health and working out our mind with engaging exercises and activities are keys to optimal memory.

Pillars of Brain Health

Many theories exist about how best to care for your brain. One research-based model by the Cleveland Clinic outlines six pillars of brain health: physical exercise, food and nutrition, medical health, sleep and relaxation, mental fitness, and social interaction. Encouragingly, substantial evidence indicates that living by these pillars may slow the progression of memory loss. For example, regular exercise, such as walking or cycling, was found to help maintain brain volume, which is one marker of brain health.

Many brain-promoting diets exist, but they all seem to share elements of the Mediterranean diet. This eating plan, focused on consuming fresh, whole fruits, vegetables, grains, and unsaturated fats, was found to be associated with better cognitive function and lower risk of cognitive impairment.

The third pillar—effectively managing medical conditions such as high blood pressure and diabetes—can provide substantial support for brain health. Even managing sensory changes such as updating prescription lenses can have a positive impact on thinking skills.

The fourth pillar—getting adequate rest and restorative sleep—is associated with better memory. The fifth pillar emphasizes the importance of cognitive reserve, meaning a stockpile of knowledge and abilities that has been found to delay the onset of dementia. Lastly, social interaction has proven useful in helping maintain aspects of cognitive functioning.

Brain Challenges

You know that feeling after you've solved a puzzle? That's your brain giving itself a little reward for being up to the challenge and successfully completing it. Our brains are wonderfully wired to respond in this way. After the reward, it gets easier to keep going, and we find ourselves up for more challenging tasks. The reverse is also true. When we don't wrestle with difficulties, our brain becomes less able to do so. The good news is that we can start small and break up tasks into smaller parts to keep our mental momentum going, and we can even have fun while we're doing it.

Some engaging ways to challenge the brain include word and number games, trivia questions, and scavenger hunts. Research has linked one type of activity with cognitive ability, called "conundrums." Conundrums involve problem-solving with novel information, such as playing chess or completing a crossword puzzle.

Games are the sweet spot for our brain. They provide a relaxed environment without stress (allowing for more creativity), as well as the concrete feedback that makes our brain crave and work toward success.

Active Engagement

It can be tempting to sit on the couch and watch television. However, our brains thrive on engagement. In fact, our creativity increases with exposure to new sights, sounds, and people, like trying an art project, conversing with someone new, or exploring different cultures. This can lend a new perspective to our understanding of the world and make our brain work to incorporate our new experience.

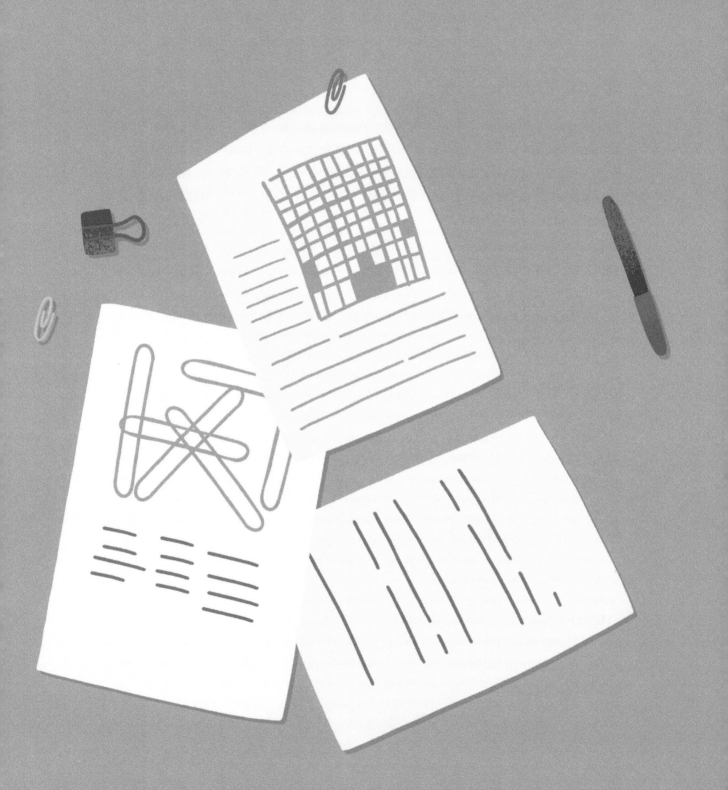

CHAPTER 2

Word Play Puzzles

Ready for some brain-boosting exercises? Let's start with word puzzles.

Word puzzles are quite popular and take many forms, from simpler ones like cryptograms, rebuses, and anagrams, to the challenging Sunday crossword.

The largest crossword ever made measured 7 feet by 7 feet and included 91,000 squares and 28,000 clues. That would be some challenge to complete! We don't have anything so daunting here, but we do offer a menu of three different types of word games to sink your teeth into: some very interesting and approachable crosswords, along with word searches and word scrambles on a variety of topics.

We've organized each set of puzzles so the easiest come first, and they get more difficult as you progress through the chapter. To help you with the puzzles, we also seeded each puzzle grid with some correct letters to serve as hints—more at the beginning of the chapter and less toward its end.

Good luck solving—and have fun!

CHALLENGE
LEVEL 1

Crosswords

People use different methods to tackle crossword puzzles, but there are some good general solving guidelines. A solid approach is to scan all the clues and the puzzle grid first. There are no strict rules here, so relax and have fun. You don't have to do all the "Across" or "Down" clues first, unless you want to. Build your foundation by filling in the answers you know right away, then solve the rest. The answers you know will inevitably fill in the crossings (or intersections) of up and down words with letters that will help you solve those, too.

To help you get started, each puzzle grid for the first six crosswords is seeded with ten letters placed in their correct position on the grid.

DAYS OF THE WEEK

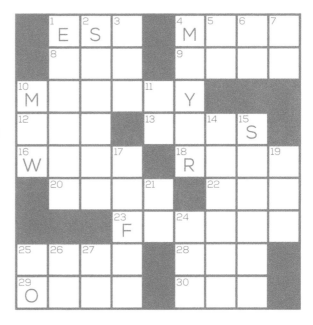

ACROSS

1. New York's time zone in the winter: Init.
4. Bright object in the sky on many nights
8. Regret
9. Big hair style
10. _____-morning quarterback (second-guesser)
12. Even's opposite
13. It is said that a rolling stone gathers none of this
16. Have on, as clothes
18. Furrows in a dirt road
20. Colorants
22. Gun group initials
23. Sgt. Joe _____ of the old-time TV series *Dragnet*
25. Chess, baseball, or Skee-Ball
28. Tree juice
29. Aroma
30. "For ___ a jolly good fellow . . ."

DOWN

1. Washed away, as soil
2. The first day of the week, when many people attend church services
3. Kennedy or Koppel
4. City bigwig
5. School __ hard knocks
6. Either's partner
7. Opposite of yes
10. Trim the grass
11. Morning time initials
14. Word for a fountain treat that sounds the same, and is spelled almost the same, as 2 Down
15. Backpack parts
17. Allude (to)
19. "O ___ can you see . . ."
21. Jr's superior
24. Suffix meaning "somewhat"
25. Stop's opposite
26. Commercial
27. Abbr. for the state in which St. Louis is located

ANSWER ON PAGE 202

BIG ANIMALS

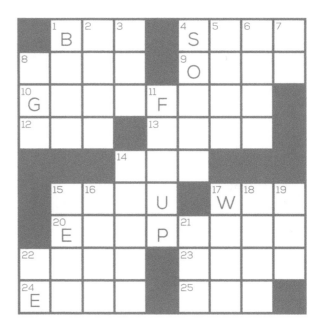

ACROSS

1. Robert, for short
4. Easy dupes
8. Descartes's "therefore"
9. Woodwind instrument
10. Large animals with very long necks
12. "___ whiz!"
13. Opposite of west
14. 6-point scores in football, for short
15. South American country where you can find llamas
17. Past tense of "is"
20. Huge gray animal with a long trunk
22. ____ *That Tune*
23. Deep black
24. Greek god of love
25. School volunteer group

DOWN

1. Soft French cheese
2. Fairy tale baddie
3. ___ constrictor (large snake)
4. Settees
5. Lincoln and Vigoda
6. The P in PM
7. Per __ (short Latin phrase meaning "in itself")
8. Main ingredient in an omelet
11. Really annoyed
14. Oak and maple, for two
15. Juicy fruit with a greenish or yellow skin
16. Sesame Street's "Tickle Me" guy
17. Desire
18. Paul ____ (1950s pop singer)
19. Pig's digs
21. In the know, to a beatnik
22. Initials for the direction opposite of southwest

ANSWER ON PAGE 202

POPULAR SPORTS

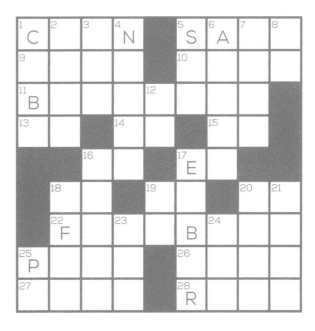

ACROSS

1. Scottish family group
5. Carpenters use these to cut wood
9. Assistant
10. Underhanded plan
11. Popular sport whose season starts with spring training in February
13. Person in their last high school year: Abbr.
14. "__ unto others as you would have them . . ."
15. Mutual __ Omaha insurance co.
16. Abbr. for "fiscal year"
17. "__ tu, Brute?"
18. Pacino or Roker
19. "__ a Yankee Doodle dandy . . ."
20. Initials for Charleston's state
22. Popular sport in which players wear helmets and shoulder pads
25. Prepare for a trip
26. One of the Great Lakes
27. Noah's boat and others like it
28. Change the decor

DOWN

1. Taxis
2. One who fibs
3. Commercials
4. Destitute, down and out
5. Health resort
6. Apportion
7. "Big bad" character in fairy tales
8. Holy person: Abbr.
12. Actress __ Derek
16. Group of sheep or birds
17. Glowing remnant of a fire
18. A long way in the distance
19. "Beat __!" ("Scram!")
20. Lost traction
21. Egyptian queen played by Liz Taylor in a film, informally
23. Approves
24. "___ you sure?"
25. Ma's mate

ANSWER ON PAGE 202

PUBLIC PLACES

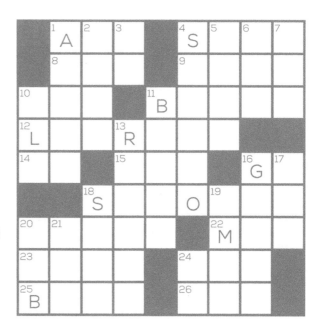

ACROSS

1. 1950s film star ___ Gardner
4. Big first for a baby
8. Obtain
9. Ripped
10. Opposite of near
11. Yogi _____ (Yankees great)
12. Public place where you can borrow books to read
14. Off's opposite
15. Dined
16. Company that's big in lighting: Init.
18. Public places where children go to be taught
20. Immerses (in liquid)
22. "Welcome" item at the front door
23. Encourage
24. Armed conflict
25. Red veggie
26. "Able was I ___ I saw Elba"

DOWN

1. Once more
2. Part of speech that describes an action being taken
3. Attorney __ law
4. Sound system that uses two or more speakers
5. In England, a supporter of the Conservative Party
6. Goof up
7. Vegetable in a pod
10. *Alice* waitress, or Progressive Insurance TV saleswoman
11. Alternatives to showers
13. Tennis _____
16. Menacing look
17. The "e" of "i.e."
18. Herb used in stuffing, or a really wise person
19. WWII General ____ Bradley
20. Underwater vessel, for short
21. Unrefined metal-bearing rock
24. You and I

ANSWER ON PAGE 202

WEATHER FORECASTS

The grid shows the following filled letters:

- 1: P
- 4: A
- 7: R
- 8 (row 2, col 4): R
- 10: S
- 15 (col 17): W
- 18: G
- 19: P
- 21: U
- 22: F

ACROSS

1. Bread with a pocket
5. Black, sticky gunk
8. *Wuthering Heights* setting
9. "Are you a man ___ ___ mouse?"
10. Nice weather forecast
12. Baseball hitter's statistic: Init.
13. He invented the lightbulb
15. Uses a thread and needle
18. Bloody
19. Jail
21. Large coffee dispenser
22. Weather forecast indicating it will be hard to see things outdoors
26. Curtain holder
27. Religious ceremony
28. Attempt
29. Adam's grandson, in the Bible

DOWN

1. Afternoon times: Init.
2. Handwritten promise to pay: Init.
3. 2,000 pounds
4. James _____, *Gunsmoke* star
5. Trunk of the human body
6. Ann _____, Mich.
7. Wet weather forecast
11. Three ft.: Abbr.
14. Disregard
15. Sudden gush
16. Mistake
17. Weather forecast good for kite-flying
20. The break __ day
23. Liquor that goes with tonic
24. '60s Pontiac muscle car: Init.
25. No's opposite

ANSWER ON PAGE 203

PEOPLE WITH PROFESSIONS

ACROSS

1. Armed conflict
4. This professional works on the stage
9. Had a meal
10. Brownish gray
11. This professional works in the operating room
13. __ masse (in a group)
14. *La Bohème* or *Aida*, e.g.
17. The Caribbean ___
19. Company name ender: Abbr.
21. Use a razor
25. Abbr. for Atlanta's state
26. This professional works in the courtroom
28. Accumulate
31. Getting on in years
32. This professional works in the cockpit
33. CIA predecessor: Init.

DOWN

1. Walks in water
2. Makes amends (for)
3. __room (where you usually find the big-screen TV)
4. At the summit of
5. Give a darn
6. "Et __, Brute?"

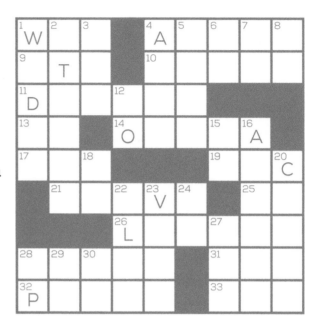

7. Photo __ (when picture-taking is permitted)
8. Musical note after Do
12. From's opposite
15. Abbr. for Providence's state
16. Heavenly beings
18. Sound of relief
20. You need these to play bridge or poker
22. In addition
23. Very, very extensive
24. Sound of disgust
27. "___-hoo" ("Anybody home?")
28. News organization: Init.
29. Musical note before fa
30. __ Capone

ANSWER ON PAGE 203

CHALLENGE
LEVEL 1

Word Searches

Word searches test our ability to find real words out of a jumble of seemingly unrelated letters. Completing word searches is great practice in deciphering patterns, keeping spelling sharp, and expanding your vocabulary.

Each word search grid has all the items in the accompanying word search list embedded in it. The word lists usually follow a theme. For instance, you can complete searches in this book focused on animals, 20th-century artists, colors, and weather. Your challenge is to spot each of these words in the grid. We've circled some letters in the grid to help you get started in your search.

There are six circled letters in each puzzle grid for this group of six easier puzzles. Each circled letter is the first letter of one of the search words. And, in these easier grids, the words read from left to right or from top to bottom. (The grids in later puzzles will get trickier, as you will see.)

THE ANIMAL KINGDOM

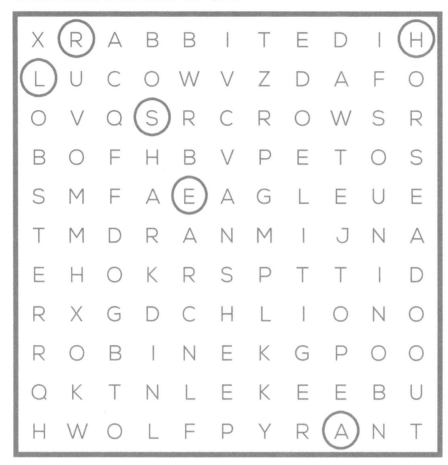

```
X  R  A  B  B  I  T  E  D  I  H
L  U  C  O  W  V  Z  D  A  F  O
O  V  Q  S  R  C  R  O  W  S  R
B  O  F  H  B  V  P  E  T  O  S
S  M  F  A  E  A  G  L  E  U  E
T  M  D  R  A  N  M  I  J  N  A
E  H  O  K  R  S  P  T  T  I  D
R  X  G  D  C  H  L  I  O  N  O
R  O  B  I  N  E  K  G  P  O  O
Q  K  T  N  L  E  K  E  E  B  U
H  W  O  L  F  P  Y  R  A  N  T
```

ANT	DOG	LOBSTER	SHEEP
BEAR	EAGLE	RABBIT	TIGER
COW	HORSE	ROBIN	WOLF
CROW	LION	SHARK	

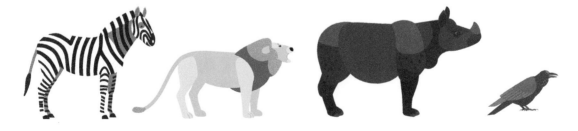

ANSWER ON PAGE 204

ROUND THINGS

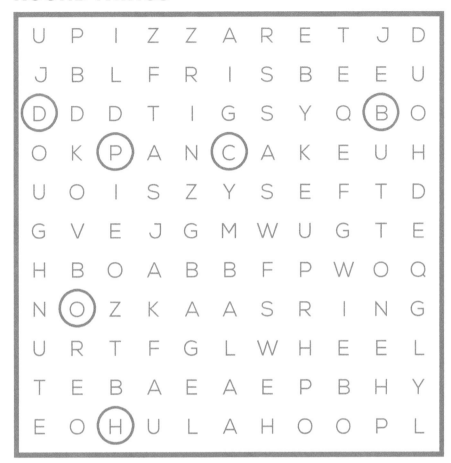

```
U  P  I  Z  Z  A  R  E  T  J  D
J  B  L  F  R  I  S  B  E  E  U
D  D  D  T  I  G  S  Y  Q  B  O
O  K  P  A  N  C  A  K  E  U  H
U  O  I  S  Z  Y  S  E  F  T  D
G  V  E  J  G  M  W  U  G  T  E
H  B  O  A  B  B  F  P  W  O  Q
N  O  Z  K  A  A  S  R  I  N  G
U  R  T  F  G  L  W  H  E  E  L
T  E  B  A  E  A  E  P  B  H  Y
E  O  H  U  L  A  H  O  O  P  L
```

BAGEL   OREO
BUTTON   PANCAKE
CYMBAL   PIE
DOUGHNUT   PIZZA
FRISBEE   RING
HULA HOOP   WHEEL

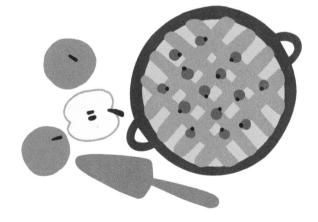

ANSWER ON PAGE 204

FOOTWEAR

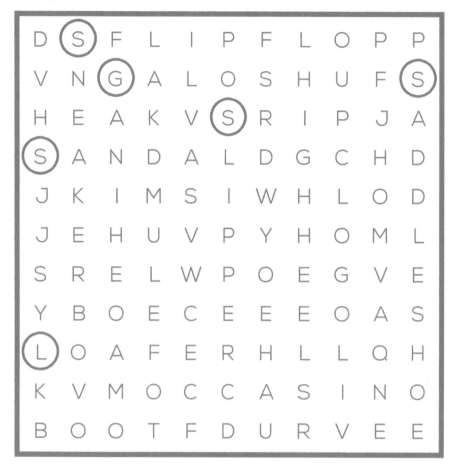

```
D  S  F  L  I  P  F  L  O  P  P
V  N  G  A  L  O  S  H  U  F  S
H  E  A  K  V  S  R  I  P  J  A
S  A  N  D  A  L  D  G  C  H  D
J  K  I  M  S  I  W  H  L  O  D
J  E  H  U  V  P  Y  H  O  M  L
S  R  E  L  W  P  O  E  G  V  E
Y  B  O  E  C  E  E  O  A  S
L  O  A  F  E  R  H  L  L  Q  H
K  V  M  O  C  C  A  S  I  N  O
B  O  O  T  F  D  U  R  V  E  E
```

BOOT
CLOG
FLIP-FLOP

GALOSH
HIGH HEELS
LOAFER

MOCCASIN
MULE
SADDLE SHOE

SANDAL
SLIPPER
SNEAKER

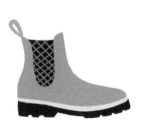
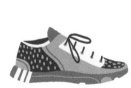
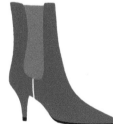
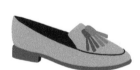

ANSWER ON PAGE 204

AT THE BEACH

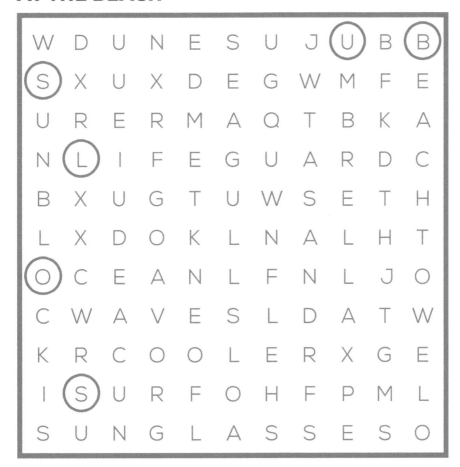

```
W  D  U  N  E  S  U  J  U  B  B
S  X  U  X  D  E  G  W  M  F  E
U  R  E  R  M  A  Q  T  B  K  A
N  L  I  F  E  G  U  A  R  D  C
B  X  U  G  T  U  W  S  E  T  H
L  X  D  O  K  L  N  A  L  H  T
O  C  E  A  N  L  F  N  L  J  O
C  W  A  V  E  S  L  D  A  T  W
K  R  C  O  O  L  E  R  X  G  E
I  S  U  R  F  O  H  F  P  M  L
S  U  N  G  L  A  S  S  E  S  O
```

BEACH TOWEL	SEAGULLS
COOLER	SUNBLOCK
DUNES	SUNGLASSES
LIFEGUARD	SURF
OCEAN	UMBRELLA
SAND	WAVES

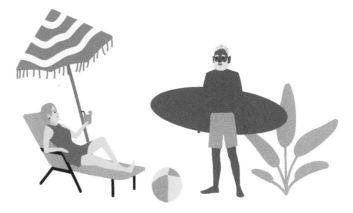

ANSWER ON PAGE 204

GAMBLING GAMES

```
B  A  C  C  A  R  A  T  E  S  S  A
L  E  G  N  C  F  P  E  I  L  G  I
A  R  O  U  L  E  T  T  E  O  I
C  X  P  O  K  E  R  M  O  T  N
K  A  K  O  A  H  K  G  L  M  R
J  F  L  O  T  T  E  R  Y  A  U
A  Q  J  C  R  C  N  F  O  C  M
C  R  A  P  S  F  O  A  I  H  M
K  R  Y  G  U  M  O  R  D  I  Y
O  M  L  O  T  T  O  O  X  N  Y
T  E  X  A  S  H  O  L  D  E  M
```

BACCARAT   LOTTO
BLACKJACK   POKER
CRAPS   ROULETTE
FARO   SLOT MACHINE
GIN RUMMY   TEXAS
KENO   HOLD 'EM
LOTTERY

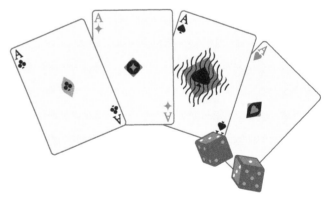

ANSWER ON PAGE 205

PARTS OF THE BODY

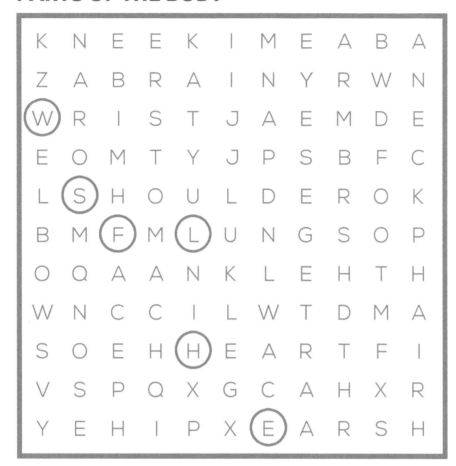

```
K  N  E  E  K  I  M  E  A  B  A
Z  A  B  R  A  I  N  Y  R  W  N
W  R  I  S  T  J  A  E  M  D  E
E  O  M  T  Y  J  P  S  B  F  C
L  S  H  O  U  L  D  E  R  O  K
B  M  F  M  L  U  N  G  S  O  P
O  Q  A  A  N  K  L  E  H  T  H
W  N  C  C  I  L  W  T  D  M  A
S  O  E  H  H  E  A  R  T  F  I
V  S  P  Q  X  G  C  A  H  X  R
Y  E  H  I  P  X  E  A  R  S  H
```

ANKLE	EYES	HIP	NOSE
ARM	FACE	KNEE	SHOULDER
BRAIN	FOOT	LEG	STOMACH
EARS	HAIR	LUNGS	WRIST
ELBOW	HEART	NECK	

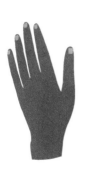
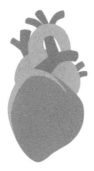

ANSWER ON PAGE 205

CHALLENGE
LEVEL 1

Word Scrambles

Like word searches, word scrambles exercise your ability to find patterns and codes in letters and words and strengthen neural pathways with the effort of rearranging letters to form real, actual words. We have two flavors of word scrambles for you to try.

The first three puzzles in this group of six easier puzzles include a list of eight words related to a specific topic. The letters have been scrambled, and you have to unscramble them! In each puzzle, we have filled in six letters that are already in their correct position in the answer.

Each of the next three puzzles presents a bit of a different challenge: You have just four mixed-up words to unscramble, but some of the letters will be in brackets, which can be combined to form another word that is the answer to a bonus question. We call these "Double Word Scrambles," and we have seeded each of these with four correctly placed letters.

WHAT'S FOR DINNER?

1. ATKES   S __ __ __ __

2. OTTAEPSO   P __ __ __ __ __ __ __

3. AESP   P __ __ __

4. RCRATSO   C __ __ __ __ __ __

5. ERBDA   __ __ __ __ __

6. URTEBT   __ __ __ __ __ __

7. DAALS   S __ __ __ __

8. ILEPPEAP   A __ __ __ __ __ __ __

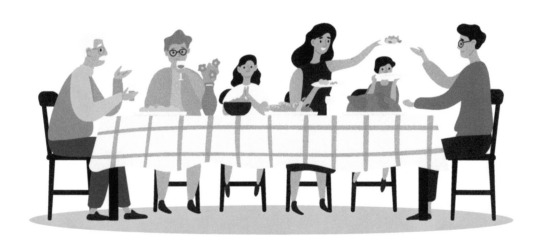

ANSWER ON PAGE 206

DO I HEAR MUSIC?

1. IONPA   P __ __ __ __
2. OLNIIV   V __ __ __ __ __
3. PHRA   __ __ __ __
4. IRGAUT   G __ __ __ __ __
5. URSMD   D __ __ __ __
6. LEFTU   __ __ __ __ __
7. PMTERUT   T __ __ __ __ __
8. OEBTORNM   T __ __ __ __ __ __

NAME THAT PRESIDENT

1. NCILNLO   L __ __ __ __ __
2. FTTA   T __ __ __
3. NIOSLW   W __ __ __ __ __
4. ARNTMU   T __ __ __ __ __
5. NDYEKNE   K __ __ __ __ __ __
6. XNNOI   __ __ __ __ __
7. RDFO   F __ __ __
8. MAAOB   __ __ __ __ __

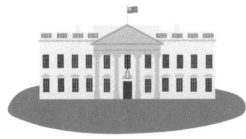

ANSWER ON PAGE 206

COLORS (DOUBLE WORD SCRAMBLE)

HOW TO SOLVE THE PUZZLE: Unscramble the letters on each line to form a word that is the name of a <u>color</u> and write the word in the grid. Then use the bracketed letters in the grids to form the word that answers the bonus question.

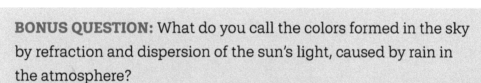

1. KNPI   P [__] [__] __

2. IWTEH   [W] __ __ __ __

3. WRNOB   [B] __ [__] __ __

4. GAEONR   O [__] [__] __ __ __

BONUS QUESTION: What do you call the colors formed in the sky by refraction and dispersion of the sun's light, caused by rain in the atmosphere?

ANSWER: __ __ __ __ B __ W

ANSWER ON PAGE 206

BIRDS (DOUBLE WORD SCRAMBLE)

HOW TO SOLVE THE PUZZLE: Unscramble the letters on each line to form a word that is the name of a <u>bird</u> and write the word in the grid. Then use the bracketed letters in the grids to form the words that answer the bonus question that follows.

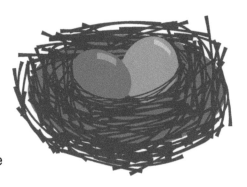

1. K D C U   [D] __ __ __

2. A L E E G   [E] __ [__] [__] __

3. E O G S O   [G] __ __ __ [__]

4. G O E I N P   P __ [__] __ [__] [__]

BONUS QUESTION: In an Aesop's fable, one of the birds listed above produced something very valuable that led to the bird's demise. Can you name that thing?

ANSWER: __ __ __ __ __   __ __ __

ANSWER ON PAGE 206

CLOTHES (DOUBLE WORD SCRAMBLE)

HOW TO SOLVE THE PUZZLE: Unscramble the letters on each line to form a word that is the name of an <u>article of clothing</u> and write the word in the grid. Then use the bracketed letters in the grids to form the word that answers the bonus question that follows.

1. S R S D E   D __ [__] __ __

2. N S P T A   [P] __ __ __ __

3. H T R I S   [S] __ __ [__] __

4. T E J C K A   J [__] __ __ [__] __

BONUS QUESTION: A colorful cloak or cape designed as a pullover that is commonly seen in Mexico is called a what?

ANSWER: __ __ __ __ __ __

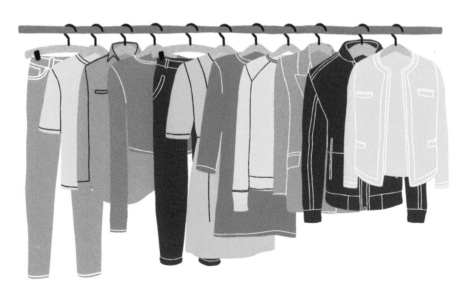

ANSWER ON PAGE 206

CHALLENGE
LEVEL 2

Crosswords

To help you get started with this next group of seven more challenging crosswords, each of the puzzle grids is seeded with eight letters placed in their correct position on the grid. The size of each crossword is also larger than the last set, increasing from 9 × 9 to 11 × 11, giving you more puzzlers to sink your teeth into.

ON THE MONEY

ACROSS

1. Another word for penny
5. Waterproof cover put over a ball field when it rains
9. Japanese luxury car brand
11. Shade of brown
12. Gin and _____
13. Mistake
14. Coffee go-with for some
16. Coin worth five pennies
19. Location
23. Historical period
24. Meadow
25. Bugle call played at army bases in the evening
27. Greenback
30. Native New Zealander
32. Handle the food for a party
35. Dodge, avoid
39. Nimble
40. "_____ Says" (child's game)
41. "The First _____" (Christmas carol)
42. Coin worth ten pennies

DOWN

1. Animal that purrs
2. Green prefix
3. Convent dweller
4. "_____ or treat!" (Halloween greeting)
5. Contract parts
6. Month between Mar. and May: Abbr.
7. Brazilian city where the 2016 Olympics were held
8. Golf score one better than bogey

CONTINUED

10. Land measurement
11. Caribbean, for one
15. Chicago transit vehicle
16. Butterfly catcher
17. 401(k) alternative
18. Soft hat with a visor
20. ___ at ease (uncomfortable)
21. Lipton or Twinings product
22. You use this to hear
26. You use your nose to
    _____ things
27. "__ as I say, not as . . ."
28. Bauxite and galena, for two
29. Hopping mad
31. "___ we there yet?"
32. Campbell's soup container
33. Gone by
34. When both teams have the
    same score, it's a ___
36. Friend, in French
37. ___ DeLuise (popular comic
    actor in the 1970s)
38. Direction opposite of
    west-southwest: Init.

ANSWER ON PAGE 207

WHAT'S STORED IN THE GARAGE?

ACROSS

1. Honey-producing insect
4. ___ Gardner (actress in *Mogambo*)
7. Money machine initials
10. ___ Thurman (actress in *Pulp Fiction*)
11. ___ Vegas, NV
12. Fem. pronoun
13. You'll find this stored in many garages
16. Bart's sister on *The Simpsons*
17. Oxidation on metal
19. Spanish word for "the"
20. Heroine of *Doctor Zhivago*
24. Gun, as an engine
25. You'll also find this stored in many garages
27. Amazement
29. Prefix for -gram or -conference
30. Urban roadway: Abbr.

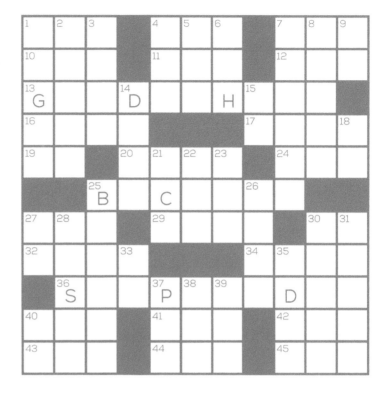

32. Strip of wood used with plaster
34. Yep's opposite
36. Another thing you'll find stored in many garages
40. Versatile vehicle, for short
41. French word for "well"
42. Bed-and-breakfast
43. ___ annum (for each year)
44. Cunning
45. Sullivan and McMahon

CONTINUED

DOWN

1. Small trumpet without valves
2. Some of it is spam
3. What we use when we listen
4. Drink similar to beer
5. Mover's vehicle
6. Residue from a fire
7. Guarantee
8. "The ones right here"
9. "__, myself, and I"
14. Surrealist painter
15. Either's partner
18. Electronic equipment found in just about every house
21. Part of a play
22. Deli bread
23. Often-injured part of the knee, for short
25. Good, _____, best
26. Extend credit
27. Gore or Pacino
28. "_____ not, want not"
30. Use money
31. Shorebirds
33. Masc. pronoun
35. *Garfield* dog
37. *Nova* network
38. Texter's chuckle
39. "___ questions?"
40. Down's opposite

ANSWER ON PAGE 207

HEALTHY THINGS TO DO

ACROSS

1. Edge
4. Taxi
7. He coaches players at a golf club
10. Wedding vow words
11. XIV × IV
12. Corn unit
13. "... ___ the land of the free ..."
14. Black gold
15. 66, e.g.: Abbr.
16. Healthy way to get exercise
19. Holiday ___ motel chain
20. Not naughty
23. Fencing swords
26. Shows the way
27. ___ Cooper cars
28. Fiddle-de-___
29. Healthy and fun way to feel better
34. 1996 Olympic torch lighter

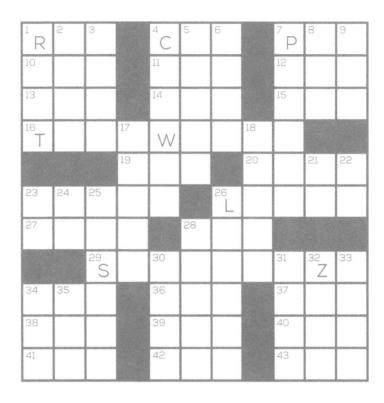

36. Campaigned (for public office)
37. Atlantic food fish
38. Tent stake
39. Three minus two
40. Bullring cheer
41. Exceedingly long time
42. Golf standard
43. A Bobbsey twin

CONTINUED

DOWN

1. Brawl
2. Brainstorm
3. Alien played by Robin Williams
4. Fright wig wearers at the circus
5. Relating to birds
6. Microsoft's ____ Gates
7. Iran, once
8. Stoolie
9. Mine product
17. "Old McDonald" refrain
18. Prepare to propose
21. It replaced the LP record: Init.
22. Letter between ar and tee
23. Aunt __ from *The Wizard of Oz*
24. Mathematical constant equal to 3.14159
25. Very junior navy officer
26. Good horseshoes throw
28. Princess ____, once married to Charles
30. Edit for size, as a photo
31. Clickable image
32. *J'accuse* author
33. Genesis locale
34. King Kong, e.g.
35. *Seinfeld* uncle

ANSWER ON PAGE 207

A MORNING RITUAL

ACROSS

1. School assistance group: Init.
4. Brazil's continent: Init.
6. Men's college social group, for short
10. Opposite of against
11. Pausing sound
12. Handed-down history
13. Having a cup of this is a morning ritual to many of us
15. Feed the kitty
16. Tehran native
18. Financial obligations
21. Some like this with their 13 Across
25. Friend, in France
26. Pilot's announcement: Init.
27. Some like this with their 13 Across
30. Piece of farm machinery used to harvest hay
32. _____ Rouge, LA
34. Saudi, e.g.
37. Some prefer this to 13 Across in the morning
41. Trim, whittle
42. Off's opposite
43. Decide to leave, with "out"
44. He and she
45. __/MAX real estate co.
46. Buddy

1 P	2	3		4	5		6 F	7	8	9
10				11			12			
13 C			14				15			
			16			17				
18	19	20				21 C		22	23	24
25								26		
27 S			28	29		30 B	31			
			32		33					
34 A	35	36			37 H			38	39	40
41					42			43		
44					45			46		

CONTINUED

DOWN

1. Army rank below corporal: Init.
2. As well
3. Dog's bark, in the comics
4. Clairvoyants
5. Type of code or rug
6. Pizzazz
7. Howard or Paul
8. Gallery display
9. Golf gadget
14. In good shape
17. Raleigh's state: Init.
18. Russian assents
19. Down Under flightless bird
20. Little's opposite
22. Slithery swimmer
23. Dined
24. Deface
28. PBS's *Downton* _____
29. Egyptian sun god
30. Daniel _____ (Kentucky pioneer)
31. Picnic pest
33. Norse thunder god
34. Appropriate
35. Cheerleader's cheer
36. Exist
38. Adjective that can precede gun, chef, or banana
39. Govt. environmental org.: Init.
40. The Braves, on the scoreboard

ANSWER ON PAGE 207

CARD GAMES

ACROSS

1. Kind of dance, or a listening device
4. Pellet gun ammo: Init.
6. Defrost
10. Pre-cable TV antenna
12. Ace in the ____ (good thing to have in reserve)
13. Trick-taking card game that developed in the 1920s
14. "Oh, woe!"
15. A few
16. Litmus reddeners
18. "___ boy!"
20. Barely get, with "out"
22. Jonah's swallower, in the Bible
25. National real estate brand
27. Always, poetically
28. Still sleeping: Archaic
30. Sufficient
32. Showy flower
36. Opera highlight
37. Card game (one that kids enjoy) where you seek to accumulate pairs of cards of the same face value
39. Suffix with mob- or gang-
40. "Tennis, _____?"
41. ["Hey, over here."]
42. Opposite of yes
43. Railway stop: Abbr.

CONTINUED

DOWN

1. Notebook projections
2. Prefix with -dynamic or -nautics
3. Straitlaced
4. Groceries container
5. Sound from a sheep
6. Bangkok native
7. Texas ___ ___ (poker variant that is very popular these days)
8. The 49th state
9. *Scream* director ___ Craven
11. Model
17. The C of TLC
19. Blue-green color
21. Former spouse, slangily
22. Plural pronoun
23. Trick-taking card game where you try to avoid cards of a certain suit
24. Hordes
26. Enlighten
29. Started
31. Auditioner's aim
33. Grande and Orinoco
34. "___ It Romantic?"
35. 1973 World Series stadium
36. Egyptian cobra
38. Lennon's lady

ANSWER ON PAGE 208

LENGTHY EVENTS

ACROSS

1. Farm building
5. ____ Cod, MA
9. Construction girder
11. One more than par
12. Rant's partner
13. Really angry
14. Very long foot race
16. Exclamation
17. Tolstoy or Durocher
18. Three feet
22. Capture
24. Holy persons: Abbr.
26. Oolong or Earl Grey
27. Famous ____ chocolate chip cookies
29. Ernie ___ (golf great)
31. Direction the opposite of NE: Init.
32. Very long TV program to raise money for a charity

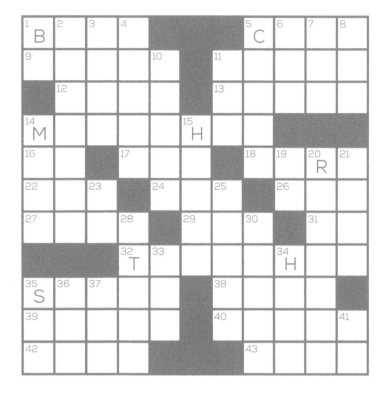

35. Thread holder
38. Impoverished
39. Use one's noodle
40. The Lone Ranger's companion
42. Heap
43. Annoyance

CONTINUED

DOWN

1. Prefix meaning "two"
2. Pres. Lincoln's first name
3. Kind of admiral
4. The "N" of U.S.N.A.
5. Like the humor on *Hee Haw*
6. Ottoman officer
7. A kitten or puppy makes a good this
8. Ogle
10. Distributes, with "out"
11. Life story, in brief
14. da Vinci's ____ *Lisa*
15. "Heartbreak ____" (Presley song)
19. Attorney __ law
20. The Homestead and The Greenbrier, for two
21. Daybreak
23. Ms. Derek
25. Caught some Z's
28. Piece of rock
30. Bend down
33. Animal with antlers
34. Sharpen
35. Fuel additive brand
36. ___ Beta Kappa
37. What Saudi Arabia produces a lot of
41. Extra playing period: Init.

ANSWER ON PAGE 208

PAPER THINGS

ACROSS

1. Makes well
6. Pas' partners
9. Verdi composition
10. Squirrel away
12. Wolf Blitzer's network: Init.
13. Papier-_____ (composite commonly made of strips of old newspapers and paste, and used in DIY art projects)
14. Paper _____ (piece of office equipment used to dispose of sensitive documents)
17. London lavatories
18. Big West Coast state: Abbr.
19. Grant's opponent during the Civil War
22. Overact
24. High-pitched and thin, as a person's voice
26. Someone on the blue end of the political spectrum: Abbr.
27. __ *Law* (1980s TV series set in a law firm)
29. Lyft competitor
30. Paper _____ (toy flier made by folding a piece of paper in the right way)
32. New Orleans footballer
35. Long, long, long time
36. Paper _____ (convenience used at many picnics)
37. *The ____ and the Ecstasy* (biographical novel about Michelangelo)
40. Japanese cash
41. Church assembly

CONTINUED

DOWN

1. Business organization, for short
2. Down's opposite
3. Where in a house the big screen TV typically is located
4. Writer _____ Hemingway
5. What a beach is made of
6. Apple's alternative to a PC
7. Cigar residue
8. Personal pronoun
10. Besmirch
11. Besmirch
14. Winter coaster
15. It is where the heart is, it is said
16. Washington, __
19. Beirut's country
20. Biblical paradise
21. Brontë's *Jane* ___
23. High society
25. Funeral tribute
28. Little Rock's state: Abbr.
30. Aardvark's morsel
31. Small green veggies
32. James Bond, for one
33. Beer's cousin
34. ___ Fleming (creator of James Bond)
38. Yes's opposite
39. Three feet: Abbr.

ANSWER ON PAGE 208

CHALLENGE
LEVEL 2

Word Searches

For this intermediate group of six word search puzzles, there are five circled letters in each puzzle grid. Each circled letter is either the spot where two embedded words intersect or (in a few cases) the first letter of one of the embedded words.

To up the challenge further, starting with this group of word searches, the words are embedded in the grid in all directions. An embedded word might have to be read from right to left, or from bottom to top, or diagonally running either up or down. So, be alert to look in all directions to see if you can locate a missing word.

POPULAR SPORTS

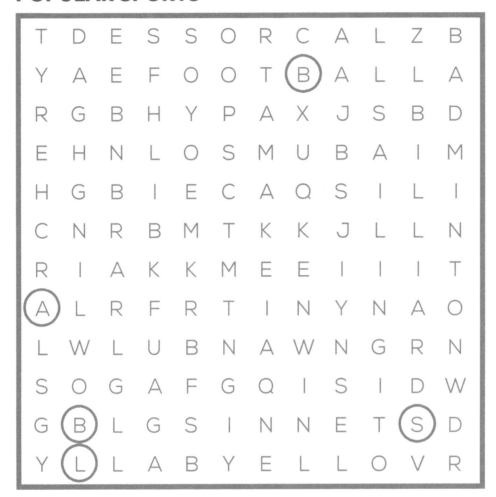

```
T D E S S O R C A L Z B
Y A E F O O T (B) A L L A
R G B H Y P A X J S B D
E H N L O S M U B A I M
H G B I E C A Q S I L I
C N R B M T K K J L L N
R I A K K M E E I I I T
(A) L R F R T I N Y N A O
L W L U B N A W N G R N
S O G A F G Q I S I D W
G (B) L G S I N N E T (S) D
Y (L) L A B Y E L L O V R
```

ARCHERY	BILLIARDS	HOCKEY	SWIMMING
BADMINTON	BOWLING	LACROSSE	TABLE TENNIS
BASEBALL	FOOTBALL	RUGBY	TENNIS
BASKETBALL	GOLF	SAILING	VOLLEYBALL

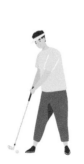
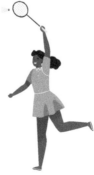
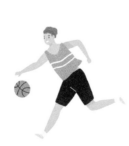

ANSWER ON PAGE 209

ON THE DANCE FLOOR

```
T  M  C  H  A  N  D  J  I  V  E  Ⓑ
U  B  O  N  Z  T  L  A  W  K  R  P
R  T  Ⓞ  H  P  X  N  P  U  E  R  T
K  Ⓦ  L  S  P  Ⓞ  B  M  A  M  O  V
E  I  A  A  S  J  H  K  A  R  V  O
Y  S  G  T  V  A  D  Y  T  S  G  F
T  T  O  P  U  A  N  X  N  N  X  R
R  L  O  U  N  S  O  O  A  N  K  U
O  Z  B  C  R  Ⓕ  I  T  V  U  U  G
T  Z  I  C  H  A  C  H  A  A  D  B
L  N  Y  I  L  A  D  A  B  M  A  L
G  L  J  I  T  T  E  R  B  U  G  K
```

BOOGALOO	CHA-CHA	JITTERBUG	TURKEY TROT
BOSSA NOVA	FOXTROT	LAMBADA	TWIST
BREAKDANCING	FRUG	MAMBO	WALTZ
BUNNY-HOP	HAND JIVE	TANGO	WATUSI

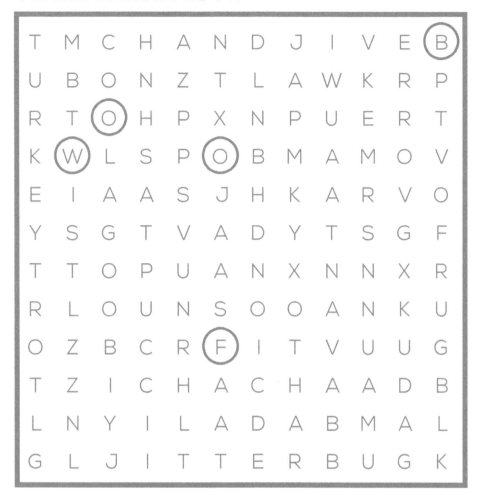

ANSWER ON PAGE 209

20TH-CENTURY ARTISTS

```
M F O S S A C I P E A D
R O I Q W K I E T M Z N
E E T W A A F N O C A B
B B G H R F R N J P I D
A M L E E O D H G D S E
S O Q E L R M D O A U K
Q Q K J I I W S E L C O
U O V A O M Z E S I N O
I W N H L D K M L R A N
A U C H A G A L L L R I
T A K C O L L O P T B N
C G I A C O M E T T I G
```

BACON	DALI	LEGER	O'KEEFFE
BASQUIAT	DE KOONING	MIRO	PICASSO
BRANCUSI	GIACOMETTI	MONDRIAN	POLLOCK
CHAGALL	KAHLO	MOTHERWELL	WARHOL

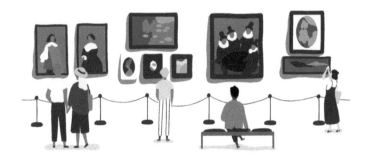

ANSWER ON PAGE 209

MODERN INVENTIONS

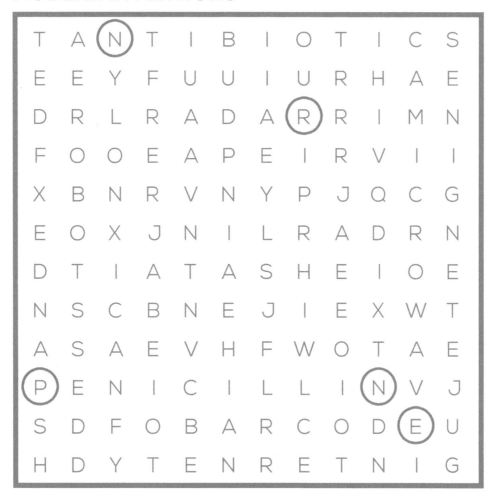

T	A	N	T	I	B	I	O	T	I	C	S
E	E	Y	F	U	U	I	U	R	H	A	E
D	R	L	R	A	D	A	R	R	I	M	N
F	O	O	E	A	P	E	I	R	V	I	I
X	B	N	R	V	N	Y	P	J	Q	C	G
E	O	X	J	N	I	L	R	A	D	R	N
D	T	I	A	T	A	S	H	E	I	O	E
N	S	C	B	N	E	J	I	E	X	W	T
A	S	A	E	V	H	F	W	O	T	A	E
P	E	N	I	C	I	L	L	I	N	V	J
S	D	F	O	B	A	R	C	O	D	E	U
H	D	Y	T	E	N	R	E	T	N	I	G

AIRPLANE	JET ENGINE	PYREX	SCANNER
ANTIBIOTICS	MICROWAVE	RADAR	SPANDEX
BARCODE	NYLON	RADIO	TEFLON
INTERNET	PENICILLIN	ROBOTS	TELEVISION

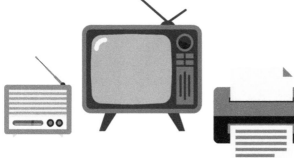

ANSWER ON PAGE 209

WHAT'S THE WEATHER LIKE TODAY?

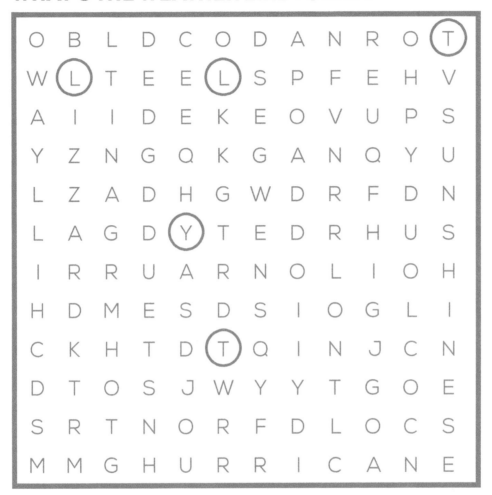

```
O B L D C O D A N R O T
W L T E E L S P F E H V
A I I D E K E O V U P S
Y Z N G Q K G A N Q Y U
L Z A D H G W D R F D N
L A G D Y T E D R H U S
I R R U A R N O L I O H
H D M E S D S I O G L I
C K H T D T Q I N J C N
D T O S J W Y Y T G O E
S R T N O R F D L O C S
M M G H U R R I C A N E
```

BLIZZARD	COLD FRONT	HEAT WAVE	SUNSHINE
CHILLY	FOGGY	HURRICANE	THUNDERSTORM
CLEAR	FROST	LIGHTNING	TORNADO
CLOUDY	GUSTY	SLEET	WINDY

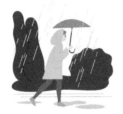 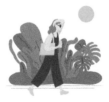 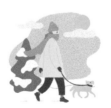 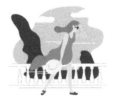

ANSWER ON PAGE 210

FOOTBALL ACTION

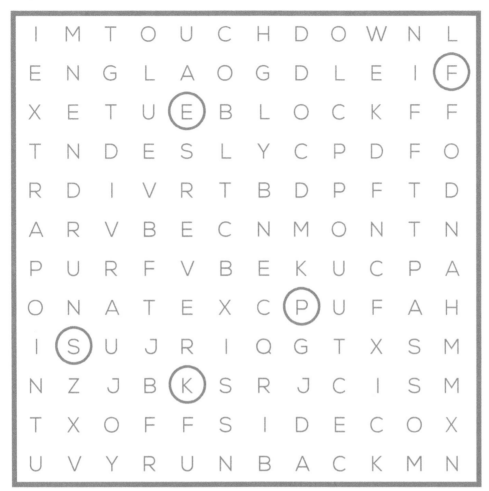

```
I  M  T  O  U  C  H  D  O  W  N  L
E  N  G  L  A  O  G  D  L  E  I  F
X  E  T  U  E  B  L  O  C  K  F  F
T  N  D  E  S  L  Y  C  P  D  F  O
R  D  I  V  R  T  B  D  P  F  T  D
A  R  V  B  E  C  N  M  O  N  T  N
P  U  R  F  V  B  E  K  U  C  P  A
O  N  A  T  E  X  C  P  U  F  A  H
I  S  U  J  R  I  Q  G  T  X  S  M
N  Z  J  B  K  S  R  J  C  I  S  M
T  X  O  F  F  S  I  D  E  C  O  X
U  V  Y  R  U  N  B  A  C  K  M  N
```

BLOCK   OFFSIDE
END RUN   PASS
EXTRA POINT   PUNT
FIELD GOAL   REVERSE
FUMBLE   RUNBACK
HANDOFF   SAFETY
INTERCEPTION   TOUCHDOWN
KICKOFF

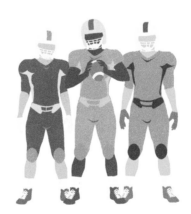

ANSWER ON PAGE 210

CHALLENGE
LEVEL 2

Word Scrambles

This group of six intermediate word scrambles gives you more of a challenge. We have added another word to each of the first puzzle types for you to unscramble and decreased the number of seeded letters.

GEMSTONES

1. NIMAODD   D __ __ __ __ __ __

2. UYRB   __ __ __ __

3. LEPRA   __ __ __ __ __

4. RDEELAM   E __ __ __ __ __ __

5. ZPOAT   __ __ __ __ __

6. AOLP   __ __ __ __

7. NSLIPE   S __ __ __ __ __

8. PIPESRAH   S __ __ __ __ __ __ __

9. HTMAYTES   A __ __ __ __ __ __

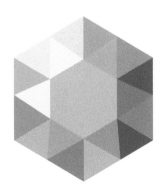
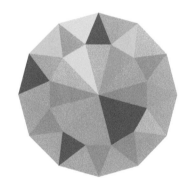
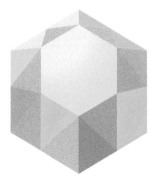

ANSWER ON PAGE 211

A HANDYMAN'S TOOLS

1. RMHEAM   H __ __ __ __ __

2. ISALN   __ __ __ __ __

3. LEPRSI   __ __ __ __ __

4. PALMC   C __ __ __ __

5. LIRLD   __ __ __ __ __

6. VLELE   __ __ __ __ __

7. RSSWCE   S __ __ __ __ __

8. HNWCRE   W __ __ __ __ __

9. PTDAETCU   D __ __ __ __ __ __ __

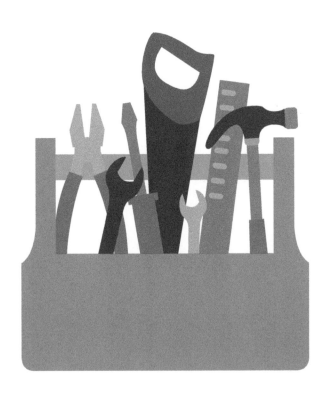

ANSWER ON PAGE 211

THIS OLD HOUSE

1. S D W O N W I   W __ __ __ __ __ __

2. S R O D O   __ __ __ __ __

3. F O R O   __ __ __ __

4. T I C A T   __ __ __ __ __

5. E R G G A A   G __ __ __ __ __

6. I S A T S R   S __ __ __ __ __

7. R P H O C   __ __ __ __ __

8. Y I H N C M E   C __ __ __ __ __

9. S T N E B M A E   B __ __ __ __ __ __ __

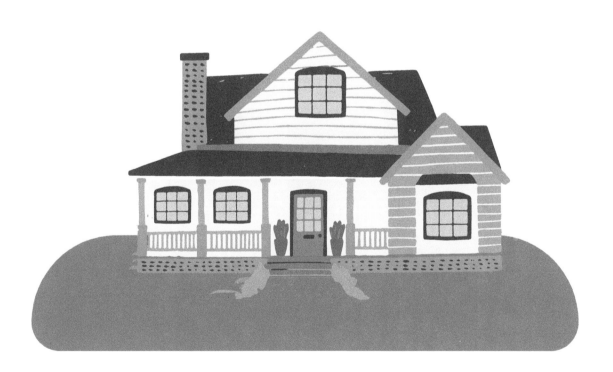

ANSWER ON PAGE 211

OFFICE SUPPLIES (DOUBLE WORD SCRAMBLE)

HOW TO SOLVE THE PUZZLE: Unscramble the letters on each line to form a word that is the name of something you'd consider an <u>office supply</u>, and write the word in the grid. Then use the bracketed letters in the grids to form the words that answer the bonus question.

1. TSAEP   [P] __ __ __ __

2. APSSTM   __ __ [__] __ [__] __

3. SERERA   E [__] __ __ [__] __

4. ECLPNI   [P] __ __ [__][__][__]

> **BONUS QUESTION:** What is the name of that ubiquitous little office gadget used to hold things together?
>
> **ANSWER:** __ __ __ __ __   __ __ __ __

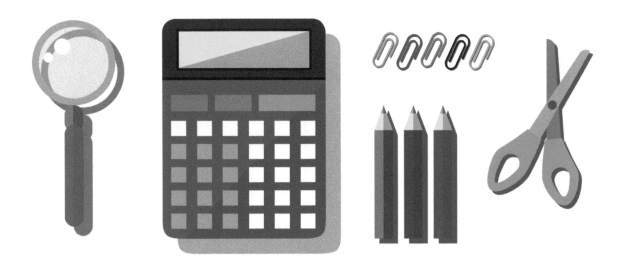

ANSWER ON PAGE 211

FLOWERS (DOUBLE WORD SCRAMBLE)

HOW TO SOLVE THE PUZZLE: Unscramble the letters on each line to form a word that is the name of a <u>flower</u> and write the word in the grid. Then use the bracketed letters in the grids to form the words that answer the bonus question.

1. Y A N S P   [__] __ __ [__] __

2. N Y E P O   P [__] [__] __ __

3. O C U S R C   C [__] __ __ [__] __

4. E O T V L I   V [__] __ [__] __ [__]

> **BONUS QUESTION:** What are the names of the two most popular flowers for weddings in the United States?
>
> **ANSWER:** (a) ___ ___ ___ ___ and (b) ___ ___ ___ ___ ___

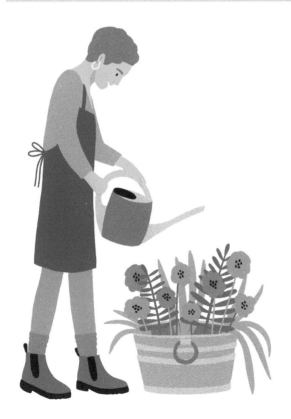

ANSWER ON PAGE 211

MAKES OF CARS (DOUBLE WORD SCRAMBLE)

HOW TO SOLVE THE PUZZLE: Unscramble the letters on each line to form a word that is a <u>make of a car</u> and write the word in the grid. Then use the bracketed letters in the grids to form the word that answers the bonus question.

1. U A R A C   [A] __ __ __ [__]

2. C B I K U   [__] [__] __ __ __

3. N O A H D   [H] __ [__] __ __

4. O T Y T A O   [T] __ __ [__] __ __

BONUS QUESTION: What is the name of the German highway system, a good portion of which has no speed limits—drivers can go as fast as they want on it?

ANSWER: __ __ __ __ __ __ __ __

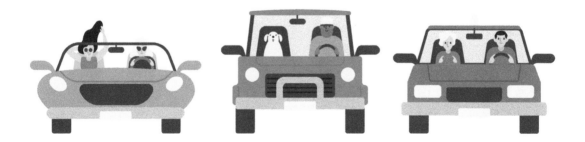

ANSWER ON PAGE 211

CHALLENGE
LEVEL 3

Crosswords

This group contains the six most difficult crosswords in the book. We still seed the puzzle grid with correctly positioned letters, but only with two to four letters. Also, the larger grid (13 × 13) makes it a bit more challenging this time. Go get 'em!

BASEBALL

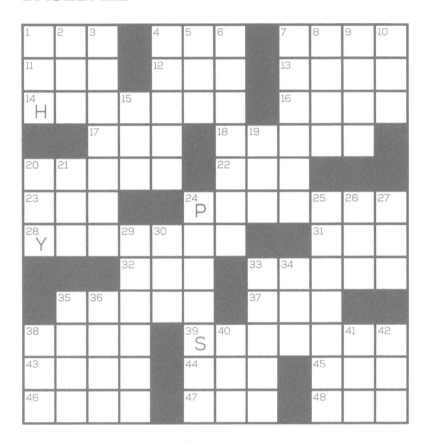

ACROSS

1. Swiss mountain
4. Excavate
7. Go with the _____ (go along with others)
11. Old French coin
12. High card
13. Assistant
14. Best hit in baseball
16. Red veggie
17. Kind of chart
18. Anagram for SNARE
20. Creates

22. ___-fi (futurist movie genre)
23. His surname was Clay, at one time
24. Baseball player who works from the mound
28. They've won more World Series than any other baseball team
31. Neighbor of Wash. and Calif.
32. "To ___ is human . . ."
33. The Mamas and the _____
35. Streamlined
37. Biblical beast of burden

38. Lose one's footing
39. "For it's one, two, three _____, you're out, at the old ball game"
43. Prod
44. Bring into play
45. Nickname for Pres. Eisenhower
46. Mimic
47. ___ thai (noodle dish)
48. Family dog, e.g.

DOWN
1. Cigar residue
2. Slang for bathroom in Britain
3. Big gourd seen on many doorsteps on Halloween
4. Challenges
5. Post-op locale: Init.
6. First book of the Bible
7. _____ softener (dryer toss-in)
8. Security for a debt
9. Lyric poems
10. Soaked
15. "Old McDonald had a farm, ___-I-O"
19. Play part
20. Month that follows April
21. Chicken ___ ___ king
24. Becomes more lively and cheerful

25. ___ ___ and jump (old term for the triple jump in the Olympics)
26. Stat for 24 Across
27. Hi-___ TV
29. Something or someone worth hanging on to
30. "Able was I ___ . . ."
33. Cut back, trimmed
34. "___ ___ was saying . . ."
35. Unappetizing food
36. Similar to
38. Health resort
40. Airport screening org.: Init.
41. Barely manage, with "out"
42. Harden

ANSWER ON PAGE 212

MOTTO

¹	²	³	■	⁴	⁵	⁶	■	⁷	⁸	⁹	¹⁰
¹¹			■	¹²			■	¹³			
¹⁴			■	¹⁵			■	¹⁶			
¹⁷O			¹⁸F			¹⁹		■			
■		²⁰		²¹			■	²²	²³	²⁴
²⁵	²⁶		■	²⁷	■	²⁸		²⁹		
³⁰		■	³¹	³²	■	³³	³⁴			
³⁵		■	³⁶		³⁷	■	³⁸			
■		³⁹A			⁴⁰		⁴¹	⁴²	
⁴³	⁴⁴	⁴⁵	■	⁴⁶			■	⁴⁷		
⁴⁸			■	⁴⁹			■	⁵⁰		
⁵¹			■	⁵²			■	⁵³		

ACROSS

1. Initials that start the names of several forensic TV series
4. Current craze
7. "____ and dandy!" ("Excellent!")
11. Possess
12. "___ Maria" (wedding air)
13. Type of history or surgery
14. Yoga class need
15. Confederate soldier, briefly
16. Entanglements
17. With 39 Across, the motto of the Three Musketeers
20. Providence's state: Init.
21. Amtrak stop: Abbr.
22. Woods's and Mickelson's org.: Init.
25. Where the buffalo roam, according to the song
28. Sheeran or Asner
29. Howard or Reagan, Jr.
30. Be in debt
31. Said twice, an informal goodbye

33. Like a chimney sweep at times
35. Wager
36. State sandwiched between Miss. and Ga.: Abbr.
38. Down's opposite
39. See 17 Across
43. "Right away!": Init.
46. Money machine initials
47. Dejected
48. More's opposite
49. Craving
50. Beginning's opposite
51. Cassette contents
52. ___ Lanka (Asian country)
53. Tofu base

25. Steal from
26. Amazement
27. And others: Abbr.
32. Puts to rest, as fears
34. Lord's Prayer start
37. Before's opposite
39. Cathedral recess
40. Prefix meaning "every"
41. Prefix meaning "a billionth"
42. Mini-whirlpool
43. Computer key
44. Last word of "America the Beautiful"
45. Nile viper

DOWN

1. Crooner Perry ____
2. Graceful aquatic bird
3. Where to find emails, sites, apps, and so on
4. Casino game
5. Asserts to be the case
6. Formal argument
7. Poultry birds
8. Anger
9. Capture
10. Chicago trains
18. ___ Newton (kind of cookie)
19. Boys
22. Asks to marry
23. Obtained
24. "___ questions?"

ANSWER ON PAGE 212

THE SILVER SCREEN

ACROSS

1. Bass or Guinness product
4. Taxi
7. "Shoo!"
11. Dover's state: Abbr.
12. Brazilian city, familiarly
13. Arizona tribe
14. "Act your ___!"
15. Chapter in history
16. Director ____ Preminger
17. Jennifer Lawrence or Brad Pitt, e.g.
20. Noah's boat
21. Happenings
25. ____ bag (type of carry-all)
27. Italian monk
28. Bard's "before"
29. "I'll take that as ___ ___"
30. ___ Cruces, NM
31. Smack
32. OPEC, e.g.
34. Washington fundraising group: Init.
35. Where 17 Acrosses can be found
39. Decorative pitcher

42. OPEC focuses on the price of this
43. Diagnostic procedure: Init.
44. Part of a skeleton
45. ET's vehicle: Init.
46. Shade tree
47. Be an omen of
48. Half a score
49. Deli bread

33. Number of feet in a yard
34. Tower supporting electric lines
36. Long prison sentence
37. Paris airport
38. Small coin
39. Recede
40. Seek the affection of
41. Conclude

DOWN

1. Eve's mate
2. Toy building block
3. Tall buildings have this in addition to stairs
4. Stream, brook
5. Broadcasts
6. Straw hats
7. Jersey _____ (popular beach area)
8. Simple bed
9. Appropriate
10. Spanish uncle
18. Choler
19. ___ Gardner (1950s 17 Across)
22. Person who just arrived
23. ___ la la
24. Area where filming is done
25. Tic-___-toe
26. ___ ___ roll (winning)
27. Residue of an atomic blast
30. Seinfeld uncle
31. Observed

ANSWER ON PAGE 212

BACK IN THE DAY

1	2	3		4	5	6		7	8	9
10		11		12				13		
14				15				16		
17 T			18				19			
		20				21			22	23	24
	25	26			27		28			
29				30		31		32		
33		34	35		36		37	38		
39				40		41				
		42 F			43			44	45	46
47	48	49			50			51		
52				53				54		
55				56				57		

ACROSS

1. Sound of a punch in the comic books
4. Mas' mates
7. Cooking measure: Abbr.
10. Lose traction
12. Egyptian snake
13. Capture
14. Identical
15. 1968 hit "Harper Valley ___"
16. The "U" in ICU
17. Back in the day, this word processor was ubiquitous in business offices. No more.
20. King: French
21. Preserve, as a body
25. Parts of children's faces great-aunts like to pinch
28. Bulgaria's capital
29. Bleacher bum's shout
30. Lincoln, familiarly
32. "___ questions?"
33. Grads

36. Measure of electrical current
39. Make fizzy
41. Plum's center
42. Back in the day, this communication device was used a lot. Not so much now.
47. Indian dress
50. A billion years
51. ____ Falco of *The Sopranos*
52. Field
53. Regret
54. Tootsie ____ candy bar
55. Obtain
56. ___ Aviv, Israel
57. ___ *Misérables*

DOWN

1. ["Hey, over here!"]
2. Approve
3. Dweeb
4. Red spice used in goulash
5. ___ Spumante (Italian sparkling wine)
6. Sudden outpouring
7. Light brown shade
8. Hit the slopes
9. Family animal
11. John ____ (big farm tractor co.)
13. Engine supercharger
18. Grief
19. Mammal has three
22. Long way off in the distance
23. Queue

24. It follows April
25. Composer ____ Porter
26. 60 minutes
27. Govt. agency that lends to start-ups: Init.
29. Lamb's sound
31. Bring together, as a jury
34. Crime syndicate
35. Amtrak stop: Abbr.
37. Photo: Abbr.
38. Early anesthetic
40. Apply, as pressure
43. Grimace or pout
44. TV's *American* ____
45. Egyptian river
46. Snakelike fishes
47. Droop
48. Exist
49. No longer working: Abbr.

ANSWER ON PAGE 212

A WALK DOWN MEMORY LANE

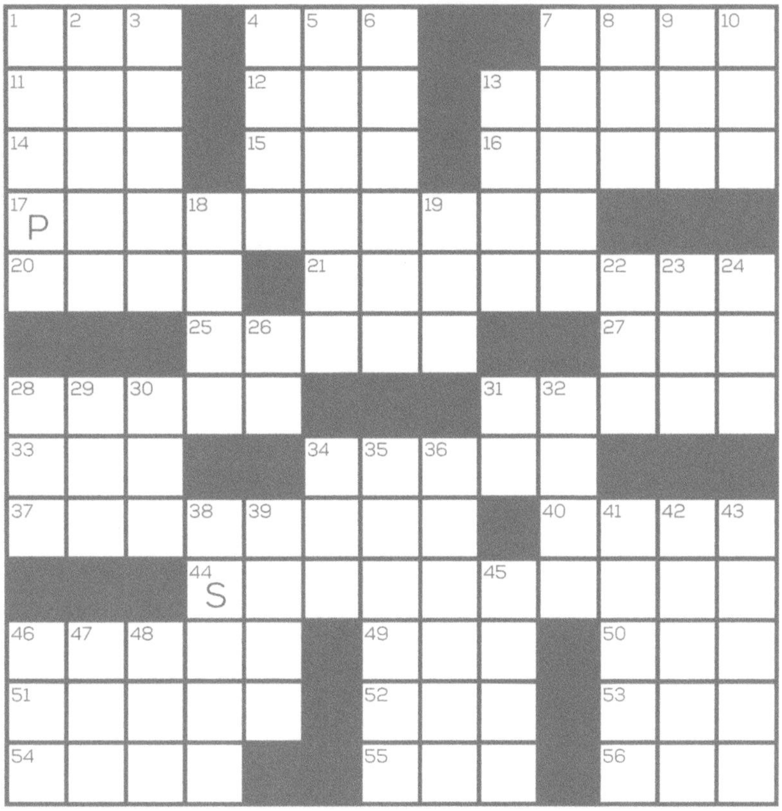

ACROSS

1. Gear tooth
4. ___ *Misérables*
7. East's opposite
11. Med. care provider: Init.
12. Crumb
13. Vietnam's capital
14. Clumsy sort
15. Sis's sibling
16. Debate
17. Leafing through this is a good way to start a walk down memory lane
20. Indian dress
21. Chews out
25. Celebratory meal
27. Prefix meaning "new" or "modern"
28. NFL _____ (where new players are selected)
31. Ewe or ram
33. School website's URL ending
34. In the know
37. Scottish musical instruments
40. ____ Parks (civil rights pioneer)

44. You can put these together to preserve good memories
46. Fine-tune
49. Actress ___ Zadora
50. Use the microwave
51. In a timid manner
52. Mork's planet
53. Summer, in Soissons
54. Ode or haiku, e.g.
55. Born, in bios
56. Lion's lair

DOWN

1. Karate blows
2. Nebraska city
3. Like a lot
4. Timber wolf
5. Printing mistakes: Lat.
6. Fur wraps
7. Heats a bit
8. High school subject: Abbr.
9. Old French coin
10. Even score
13. Tote
18. Minor quarrel
19. Short order sandwich initials
22. "We're number ___!"
23. Lawyer's charge
24. Dandy
26. "___ tu, Brute?"
28. Cotillion girl
29. Nutritional information: Abbr.

30. Month between Jul. and Sept.: Abbr.
31. Last year in high school: Abbr.
32. Medal of Honor recipient
34. Month between Mar. and May: Abbr.
35. Gun or sword, e.g.
36. Aim (with "to")
38. Sacred song
39. Gross, offensive
41. Seeped
42. Fly on ice
43. Colorado skiing mecca
45. Cook in the oven
46. Recipe abbreviation
47. Reporter's question
48. Hurricane's center

ANSWER ON PAGE 213

SUNNY SIDE UP

ACROSS

1. Mars, to the Greeks
5. Rock concert equipment
8. Apple product
12. Plumbing problem
13. Whopper
14. Entryway
15. Pessimist's opposite
17. Catch sight of
18. Dawn goddess
19. Bigheadedness
20. Mai ___ (rum cocktail)
21. Corral
22. Smallest state: Init.
23. Three, in Italy
26. Friars Club event
29. Public sale to the highest bidder
31. Sciences' partner
32. Wager
33. Roman poet
34. Frontiersman
36. Detects by touching
37. Hawaiian dish
38. Off's opposite
39. ___ Angeles, CA

40. Child's game
42. Knight's title
43. Motorist's org.: Init.
46. McCartney or Rudd
48. What a 15 Across usually is
50. Assistant
51. French word of approval
52. Word repeated after "Que," in song
53. Cedar or elm, e.g.
54. "Send help!" initials
55. "___ the night before . . ."

DOWN

1. Hand cream ingredient
2. Seized vehicle, for short
3. Dines
4. Hit the slopes
5. True up
6. Japanese soup
7. Favorite
8. Bright thought
9. With 28 Down, what a 15 Across has
10. "Alley ___!"
11. Like some martinis
16. Run into
20. Twitch
21. ["Hey, over here!"]
22. Groove in a dirt road
24. Stir up
25. Breaks off
26. Coarse file

27. Popular cookie brand
28. See 9 Down
29. ___ Lingus (Irish carrier)
30. "Little piggies"
32. London's Big ___
35. Sleep like a ___
36. Golfer's shout
39. Property claims
41. Away from the wind
42. "Git!"
43. Not many
44. Heavenly glow
45. "Oh, woe!"
46. Frisk, with "down"
47. Broadcast
48. TV network: Init.
49. Alphabet run starting after Q

ANSWER ON PAGE 213

CHALLENGE
LEVEL 3

Word Searches

In this group of the six most challenging word search puzzles in the book, the four circled letters in each puzzle grid represent letters that are parts of embedded search words. Once again, we've increased the size of the grid a notch to make the embedded words a tad harder to find. Happy hunting!

CAR PARTS

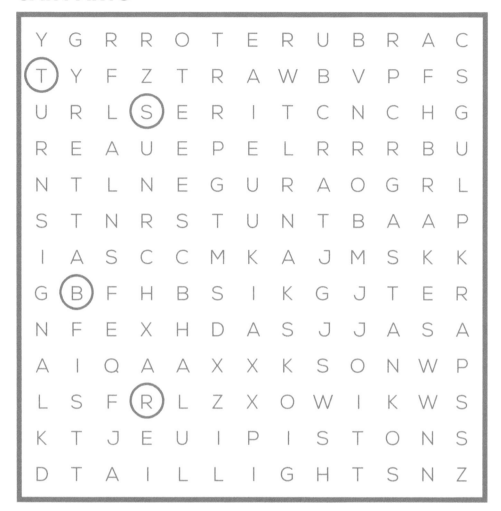

```
Y  G  R  R  O  T  E  R  U  B  R  A  C
T  Y  F  Z  T  R  A  W  B  V  P  F  S
U  R  L  S  E  R  I  T  C  N  C  H  G
R  E  A  U  E  P  E  L  R  R  R  B  U
N  T  L  N  E  G  U  R  A  O  G  R  L
S  T  N  R  S  T  U  N  T  B  A  A  P
I  A  S  C  C  M  K  A  J  M  S  K  K
G  B  F  H  B  S  I  K  G  J  T  E  R
N  F  E  X  H  D  A  S  J  J  A  S  A
A  I  Q  A  A  X  X  K  S  O  N  W  P
L  S  F  R  L  Z  X  O  W  I  K  W  S
K  T  J  E  U  I  P  I  S  T  O  N  S
D  T  A  I  L  L  I  G  H  T  S  N  Z
```

AXLE
BATTERY
BRAKES
CARBURETOR
CLUTCH
CRANKSHAFT
GAS TANK
GAUGES
PISTONS

RADIATOR
SPARK PLUGS
TAILLIGHTS
TIRES
TRANSMISSION
TURN SIGNAL
WIPERS

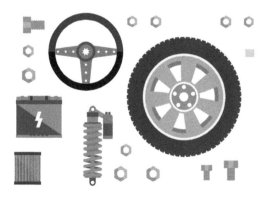

ANSWER ON PAGE 214

COLORFUL COLORS

```
T R J N C R I M S O N H P
U Y E J A B X Z X E D U N
B K Y V V V D D R G R O E
U E U L L H Y U S P W M E
R T V C J I Z B L R A A R
N O B U E A S E L S Q G G
T G C H A R T R E U S E T
O I T E S M U A O S E N S
R D Q U R P G L A L F T E
A N B S I I C E E H W A R
N I H N O F S O Q A M H O
G S K W O L L E Y F N O F
E W W C E N I R E G N A T
```

AZURE
BURNT ORANGE
CERISE
CERULEAN
CHARTREUSE
CRIMSON
FOREST GREEN
INDIGO
MAGENTA

MAUVE
NAVY BLUE
PINK
PURPLE
SILVER
TANGERINE
YELLOW

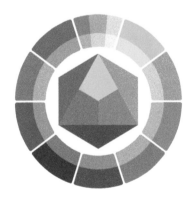

ANSWER ON PAGE 214

POCKET FULL OF POSIES

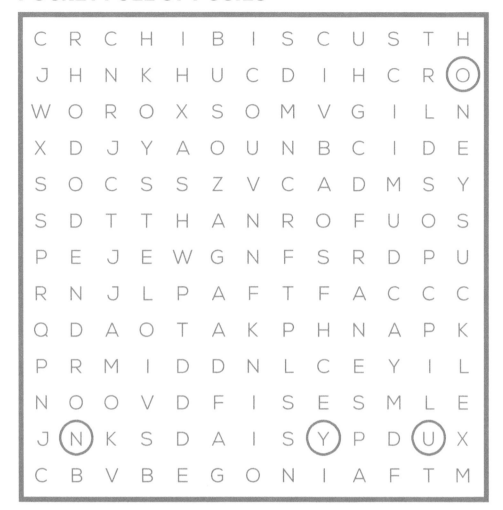

```
C  R  C  H  I  B  I  S  C  U  S  T  H
J  H  N  K  H  U  C  D  I  H  C  R  O
W  O  R  O  X  S  O  M  V  G  I  L  N
X  D  J  Y  A  O  U  N  B  C  I  D  E
S  O  C  S  S  Z  V  C  A  D  M  S  Y
S  D  T  T  H  A  N  R  O  F  U  O  S
P  E  J  E  W  G  N  F  S  R  D  P  U
R  N  J  L  P  A  F  T  F  A  C  C  C
Q  D  A  O  T  A  K  P  H  N  A  P  K
P  R  M  I  D  D  N  L  C  E  Y  I  L
N  O  O  V  D  F  I  S  E  S  M  L  E
J  N  K  S  D  A  I  S  Y  P  D  U  X
C  B  V  B  E  G  O  N  I  A  F  T  M
```

ASTER

BEGONIA

CARNATION

CHRYSAN-
  THEMUM

CROCUS

DAFFODIL

DAHLIA

DAISY

HIBISCUS

HONEYSUCKLE

ORCHID

PANSY

RHODODENDRON

ROSE

TULIP

VIOLET

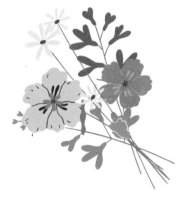

ANSWER ON PAGE 214

2019 NCAA "SWEET SIXTEEN" TEAMS

```
M  M  E  (E) S  S  E  N  N  E  T  T  A
(H) I  I  A  U  B  U  R  N  Y  X  (N) F
C  C  C  C  E  D  I  Q  O  M  I  O  L
E  A  E  H  H  M  R  R  F  L  G  T  O
T  I  C  T  I  I  E  U  O  P  H  G  R
S  N  N  G  A  G  G  R  P  G  V  N  I
A  I  R  F  O  I  A  A  O  C  O  I  D
X  G  U  N  R  C  N  N  T  Q  H  A
E  R  Y  Y  H  B  Z  I  S  U  X  S  S
T  I  I  T  T  A  I  U  G  T  I  A  T
G  V  R  K  G  I  O  K  M  R  A  W  A
D  O  G  A  S  H  E  K  U  D  I  T  T
N  B  L  K  E  N  T  U  C  K  Y  V  (E)
```

AUBURN	NORTH
DUKE	CAROLINA
FLORIDA	OREGON
STATE	PURDUE
GONZAGA	TENNESSEE
HOUSTON	TEXAS TECH
KENTUCKY	VIRGINIA
MICHIGAN	VIRGINIA TECH
MICHIGAN	WASHINGTON
STATE	

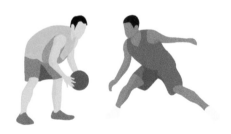

ANSWER ON PAGE 214

SYNONYMS FOR "CAREFUL"

```
A   Z   S   U   O   I   T   U   A   C   L   P   S
L   P   W   A   R  (Y)  T   Q   H   I   R   S   U
U   K   A   V   G   H   S   E   H   U   I   C   O
F   D   Z   I   R   U   E   S   D   I   M   R   L
I   O   T   A   N   D   A   E   U   T   J   U   U
T   D   R   T   F   S   N   R   E   F   X   P   C
U   P   E   U   C   T   T   E   D   U   T   U   I
(D)  E   L   I   B   E  (R)  A   T   E   V   L   T
H   Y   X   Z   D   C   D   F   K   F   D   O   E
B   R   M   A   S   U   U   Z   A   I   T   U   M
W   A   L   I   C   B   T   G   J   O   N   S   H
H   H   D   Q   Y   T   S   S   Y   V   T   G   X
T  (C)  E   P   S   M   U   C   R   I   C   C   Z
```

CAUTIOUS	DISCREET	GUARDED	PRUDENT
CHARY	DUTIFUL	HEEDFUL	SCRUPULOUS
CIRCUMSPECT	EXACT	METICULOUS	STUDIED
DELIBERATE	FUSSY	PAINSTAKING	WARY

ANSWER ON PAGE 215

THE 15 LARGEST STATES, AND THE SMALLEST STATE (BY AREA)

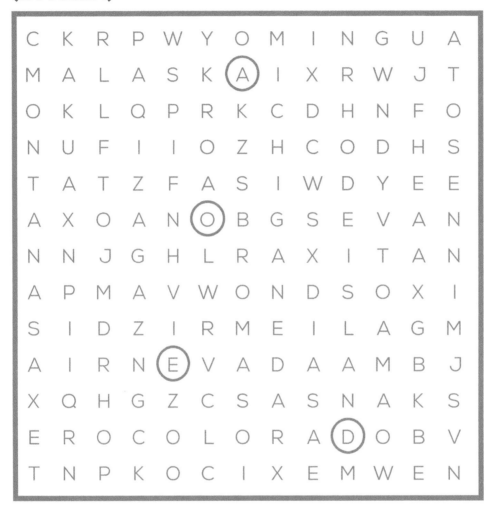

ALASKA (#1: 663,300 sq. mi.)
ARIZONA (#6: 113,998 sq. mi.)
CALIFORNIA (#3: 163,696 sq. mi.)
COLORADO (#8: 104,185 sq. mi.)
IDAHO (#14: 83,642 sq. mi.)
KANSAS (#15: 82,277 sq. mi.)
MICHIGAN (#11: 96,716 sq. mi.)
MINNESOTA (#12: 86,943 sq. mi.)
MONTANA (#4: 147,040 sq. mi.)

NEVADA (#7: 110,567 sq. mi.)
NEW MEXICO (#5: 121,697 sq. mi.)
OREGON (#9: 98,466 sq. mi.)
RHODE ISLAND (#50: 1,212 sq. mi.)
TEXAS (#2: 269,597 sq. mi.)
UTAH (#13: 84,899 sq. mi.)
WYOMING (#10: 97,818 sq. mi.)

ANSWER ON PAGE 215

CHALLENGE
LEVEL 3

Word Scrambles

In this group of six hard word scrambles, we've once again added another word to each of the first puzzle type for you to unscramble. We've decreased the number of seeded letters even more. Enjoy the added challenge.

GREEN VEGGIES

1. E Y C R L E   __ __ __ __ __ __
2. V D E I N E   __ __ __ __ __ __
3. E L K A   __ __ __ __
4. A C B E B G A   __ __ __ __ __ __ __
5. E T L C U E T   __ __ __ __ __ __ __
6. E S A Y R P L   __ __ __ __ __ __
7. U U A G L R A   A __ __ __ __ __ __
8. U U M R B C E C   C __ __ __ __ __ __ __
9. O R I L C B O C   B __ __ __ __ __ __ __
10. H U C Z I I C N   Z __ __ __ __ __ __ __

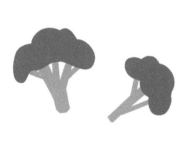
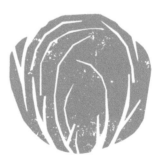

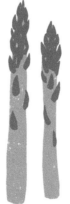
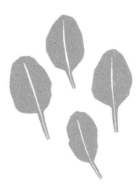

ANSWER ON PAGE 216

EASTERN U.S. STATES

1. METROVN   __ __ __ __ __ __ __
2. NAEMI   __ __ __ __ __
3. IOOH   __ __ __ __
4. DRLAOIF   __ __ __ __ __ __ __
5. AALMBAA   __ __ __ __ __ __ __
6. AREIOGG   __ __ __ __ __ __ __
7. DNAIAIN   I __ __ __ __ __ __
8. DYMRANLA   M __ __ __ __ __ __ __
9. YKETCNKU   K __ __ __ __ __ __ __
10. HNMAICGI   M __ __ __ __ __ __ __

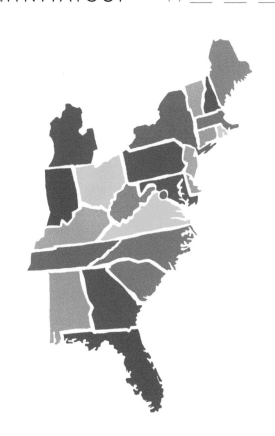

ANSWER ON PAGE 216

TOP U.S. COLLEGES

1. ADHVRRA   __ __ __ __ __ __ __

2. YMERO   __ __ __ __ __

3. EYLA   __ __ __ __

4. WRNBO   __ __ __ __ __

5. LNCERLO   __ __ __ __ __ __ __

6. GSUETRR   __ __ __ __ __ __ __

7. TNROPNIEC   P __ __ __ __ __ __ __ __

8. MLACIUBO   C __ __ __ __ __ __ __

9. OAFTDSNR   S __ __ __ __ __ __ __

10. MHDUROATT   D __ __ __ __ __ __ __ __

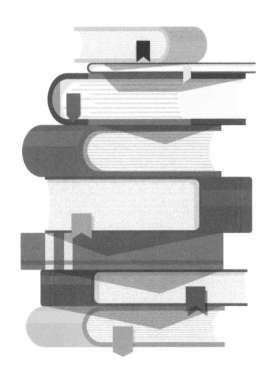

ANSWER ON PAGE 216

TREES (DOUBLE WORD SCRAMBLE)

HOW TO SOLVE THE PUZZLE: Unscramble the letters on each line to form a word that is the name of a <u>tree</u> and write the word in the grid. Then use the bracketed letters in the grids to form the word that answers the bonus question.

1. D R E A C   __ __ [__] __ __

2. O W W L L I   [__] __ __ __ [__] __

3. C R P E S U   S __ [__] __ __ [__]

4. O W G D D O O   D __ __ __ [__] __ [__]

BONUS QUESTION: What is the name of the California tree that lives a very long time and grows the tallest of any tree on earth?

ANSWER: __ __ __ __ __ __ __

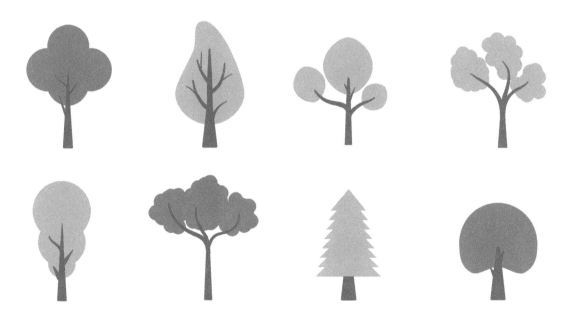

ANSWER ON PAGE 216

BIRDS (DOUBLE WORD SCRAMBLE)

HOW TO SOLVE THE PUZZLE: Unscramble the letters on each line to form a word that is the name of a <u>bird</u> and write the word in the grid. Then use the bracketed letters in the grids to form the word that answers the bonus question.

1. K T S R O ⎯⎯ [⎯⎯] ⎯⎯ [⎯⎯] ⎯⎯

2. I C N H F ⎯⎯ [⎯⎯] ⎯⎯ [⎯⎯][⎯⎯]

3. L W W S O A L S ⎯⎯ ⎯⎯ ⎯⎯ ⎯⎯ [⎯⎯] ⎯⎯

4. G A L E L S U [S] ⎯⎯ ⎯⎯ ⎯⎯ ⎯⎯ ⎯⎯ ⎯⎯

BONUS QUESTION: What is the name of the African bird that grows to be the largest of all birds? Big ones can weigh over 340 pounds.

ANSWER: ⎯⎯ ⎯⎯ ⎯⎯ ⎯⎯ ⎯⎯ ⎯⎯

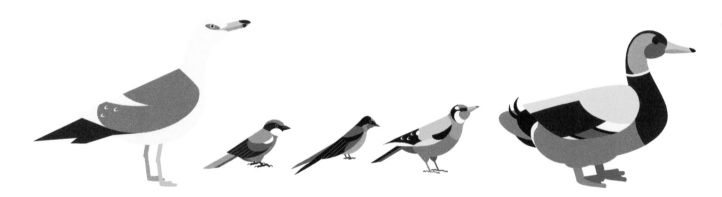

ANSWER ON PAGE 216

UNITED NATIONS MEMBER COUNTRIES (DOUBLE WORD SCRAMBLE)

HOW TO SOLVE THE PUZZLE: Unscramble the letters on each line to form a word that is the name of a <u>United Nations member country</u> and write the word in the grid. Then use the bracketed letters in the grids to form the words that answer the bonus question.

1. D E S N E W   [__] __ __ [__] __ __

2. I K A T W U   __ [__] __ [__] __ __

3. N A S E I O T   E [__][__][__] __ __ __

4. Y G H R N U A   [H][__][__] __ __ __ __

BONUS QUESTION: What is the name of the African country that became the 193rd (and newest) member-state of the United Nations in 2011?

ANSWER: __ __ __ __   __ __ __ __ __

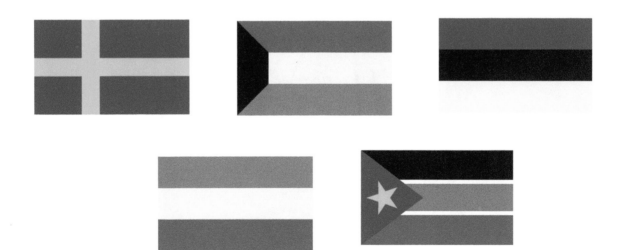

ANSWER ON PAGE 216

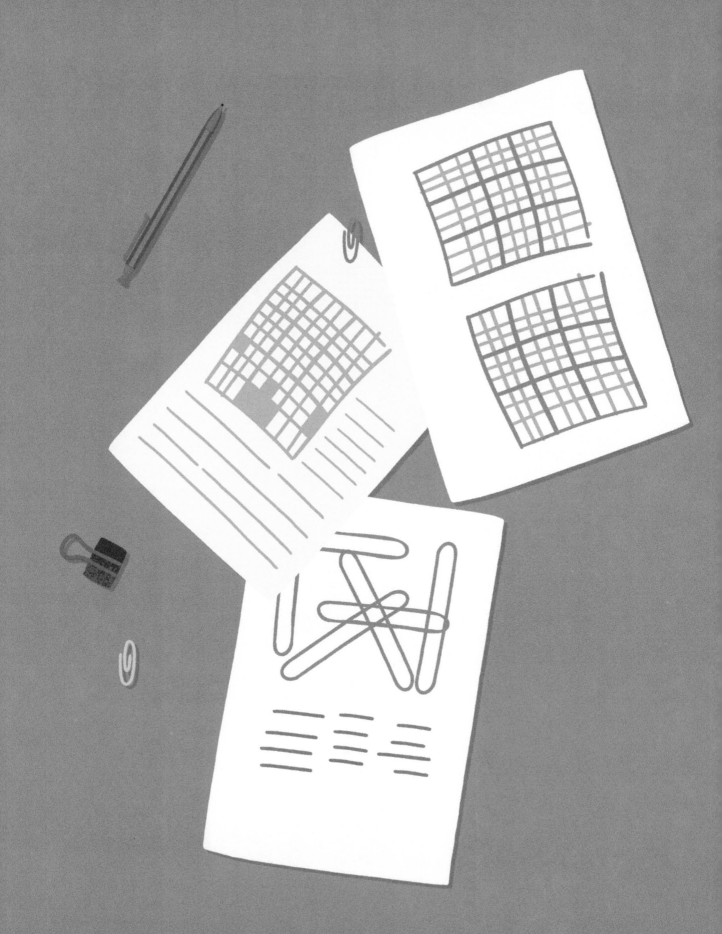

CHAPTER 3

By the Numbers Puzzles

Humans have been using numbers for at least 5,000 years. In Western societies, we used Roman numerals until the 14th century, when we switched to the Arabic numbering system that we still use today.

The thing about numbers is that they are so useful in just about every aspect of life, from commerce to science to the more mundane tasks, like keeping track of pocket change, grocery bills, and sale discounts. It's not surprising, then—given how much we love games—that we have incorporated numbers into all sorts of games.

This chapter offers you three types of number games to play—Sudokus, number searches (similar to the word searches in chapter 2), and number fill-ins using a crossword grid.

You will find 45 number puzzles here, organized with the easiest puzzles first, giving way to more challenging puzzles as you progress through the chapter.

CHALLENGE
LEVEL 1

Sudokus

To solve a Sudoku puzzle, your challenge is to fill each empty cell with a number from 1 through 9 so that each row across, each column down, and each 3 × 3 "cage" contains all the numbers 1 through 9, without repeats.

SUDOKU 1

9			1		3			4
1	6		4			7	3	5
		2		8	7			1
		1		7				8
8	4		2		5		6	3
6				4		2		
7			9	5		3		
3	8	6			4		5	9
5			6		8			2

SUDOKU 2

1	5		9	6	2	7		
	4				5			
6		8				1	9	
2	6	1	5		8			
8	7		1	2	3		5	4
			6		7	8	1	2
	9	5				4		1
			4				8	
		6	7	5	1		2	9

ANSWER ON PAGE 217

SUDOKU 3

2					4	9		
4		5			9			1
1	8		6	3		5		2
		4			1			8
	5	1	3		6	7	9	
7			8			3		
9		8		6	3		2	5
6			4			8		9
		3	1					7

SUDOKU 4

2	4		3	8		1		7
5		3		7			2	4
7		1	6	4		9		
2					7		4	
			5		4			
	7		8					6
		7		5	6	4		3
3	9			1		7		5
4		6		3	9		8	

ANSWER ON PAGE 217

SUDOKU 5

4		6		9		1	3	
					6		5	7
3	7	8			1	9		
			7		9	5		
7								6
		1	3		4			
		5	6			3	4	1
2	3			1				
	1	4		5		7		8

ANSWER ON PAGE 218

CHALLENGE
LEVEL 1

Number Searches

Like word search puzzles, the number search puzzle grid has all the items in the search list embedded in it. Your job is to spot these items in the grid. We've circled some digits on the grid to help you get started in your search. There are six circled digits in each puzzle grid for this group of five easier puzzles. Each circled digit is the first digit of one of the embedded numbers or the spot where two embedded numbers intersect. In these easier grids, the embedded numbers read from left to right, or from top to bottom.

Note that some embedded numbers might intersect with other embedded numbers—a horizontal number could cross a vertical number. And, in the first puzzle on the next page, we have located one of the embedded numbers for you by circling it on the grid and scratching it off the list of embedded numbers to be located.

NUMBER SEARCH 1

```
3  6  7  5  9  2  1  2  8  3 (5)
0 (4) 8  0  7  6  8  5  4  1  5
7  0  6  5  8  7  6 (3) 5  6  4
8  3  8  6  1  2  3  1  7  9  8
1  3  4  4  8 (6  5  4  3  2) 7
(2) 0  8  5  5  5  3  5  3  0  6
7  3  4  6  1  7  8  9  7  3  2
3  3  1  9  2  5  7  3  8  8  1
3  6  7  1  2  9  4  5  3  7  5
4 (8) 3  5  1  3  7  5  2  2  0
8  5  9 (9) 7  5  8  0  6  8  6
```

1221	4807685	555	7065
273348	50564	~~65432~~	835137522
3145935	55487	6848417	97580686

ANSWER ON PAGE 218

NUMBER SEARCH 2

```
6  8  2  7  3  7  4  7  5  6  7
0  5  6  5  1  6  8  0  2  3  3
0  8  5  9  3  9  2  6  7  5  4
3  0  3  5  2  3  6  8  7  4  6
2  3  9  9  4  1  5  6  8  0  7
3  2  0  2  9  1  6  7  2  6  8
6  4  8  1  7  2  3  2  0  9  5
6  3  3  2  1  0  9  3  7  2  4
8  2  1  3  0  4  6  0  4  3  6
2  6  7  8  3  3  9  3  4  4  0
8  1  0  1  0  1  7  5  6  4  2
```

10101	32095	440	734678
132497	3321	6003	7693112
2737475	354069	65390	82130460

ANSWER ON PAGE 218

NUMBER SEARCH 3

```
9  5  5  6  7  2  3  2  1  2  3
5  4  2  1  3  4  8  4  4  0  1
0  5  8  3  1  8  4  5  6  0  5
0  5  3  3  0  4  1  3  9  2  2
6  8  3  6  9  9  4  3  0  3  5
7  7  2  9  2  3  6  7  8  4  2
8  9  4  6  1  4  5  3  1  9  4
6  9  5  4  6  7  4  5  6  5  9
3  0  8  2  5  8  3  4  5  5  3
2  7  7  1  0  1  0  1  3  5  4
0  2  7  5  3  2  5  3  4  6  8
```

10101	4401	55672321	695467
234955	500678	58345	7310921
337	525249348	6320	7532534

ANSWER ON PAGE 219

NUMBER SEARCH 4

```
7  3  7  4  6  7  2  8  9  6  9
9  2  6  0  0  5  4  1  5  5  9
4  2  7  8  1  8  4  5  1  7  7
8  7  3  3  3  4  0  8  4  3  3
5  9  4  6  0  6  5  7  7  8  4
5  6  1  7  6  3  5  7  1  5  5
6  3  2  1  6  2  6  5  0  7  6
3  8  3  4  3  5  7  1  1  4  6
2  9  6  2  3  3  9  3  0  6  3
7  7  4  4  1  6  2  4  5  4  9
3  8  5  0  2  7  1  9  7  4  5
```

123645	41624	59460657	6633
3334	5367	600541	9485563
37467289	573857464	65076	997345

ANSWER ON PAGE 219

NUMBER SEARCH 5

```
6  6  7  4  9  0  2  5  9  3  9
1  8  3  7  2  0  0  7  1  2  3
0  2  9  8  1  6  1  4  2  7  2
6  5  2  1  7  2  3  8  8  9  2
9  5  3  7  5  1  3  5  7  9  8
7  2  8  1  7  5  0  8  1  6  3
1  5  7  4  0  8  6  7  9  8  4
8  1  5  8  1  4  3  9  0  3  5
5  7  3  1  9  2  5  1  4  0  3
4  7  8  1  0  9  6  2  7  5  1
8  1  6  1  6  5  3  7  3  3  4
```

111	392387	5939	7334
13579	48587	6674902	93228345
200712	5814390	68305	
29816	584295	69718548	

ANSWER ON PAGE 219

CHALLENGE
LEVEL 1

Number Fill-Ins

Number fill-in puzzles make fun use of a crossword grid to challenge you to take the large group of numbers in the fill-in list and add them to the grid. Your goal is to have all numbers placed in the grid, fill all the cells in the grid, and have each number align perfectly with the numbers that cross it. We have placed one number where it belongs in the grid to get you started.

   Sounds like a challenge, doesn't it? It is, but it can be done by using deductive logic and taking things one step at a time. Look at one slot in the grid where you already know what one of the digits is and where it should be. Then search through the numbers in the list to find the only number that can fit that slot. Once you have found it, pencil it in. Then look for another slot in the grid that has at least one digit already filled in and see if you can find the number that fits it. Build out from there.

NUMBER FILL-IN 1

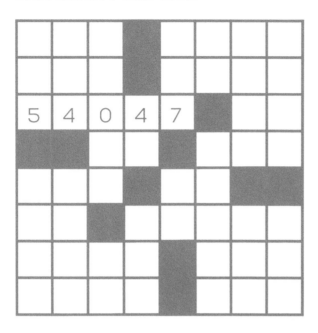

TWO DIGITS
24
32
39
49
54
57
67
77

THREE DIGITS
217
294
321
385
535
554
659
734
823
890
925
954

FOUR DIGITS
1243
2345
2349
4465
5783
5823
9379
9752

FIVE DIGITS
10034
54897
67885

ANSWER ON PAGE 220

NUMBER FILL-IN 2

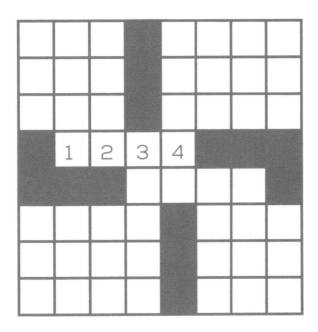

THREE DIGITS	FOUR DIGITS	FIVE DIGITS
248	1078	37582
316	2435	71346
353	3748	
356	4578	
376	5711	
407	6762	
455	7445	
474	7689	
496	8457	
505	8562	
577	9905	
588		
654		
754		

ANSWER ON PAGE 220

NUMBER FILL-IN 3

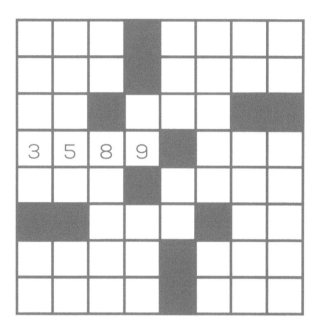

TWO DIGITS	THREE DIGITS	FOUR DIGITS	FIVE DIGITS
12	130	1451	25356
13	340	1650	45147
19	347	4183	47634
33	425	8653	61036
36	468	9678	70208
54	573		88575
58	678		
63	754		
64	781		
91	843		

ANSWER ON PAGE 220

NUMBER FILL-IN 4

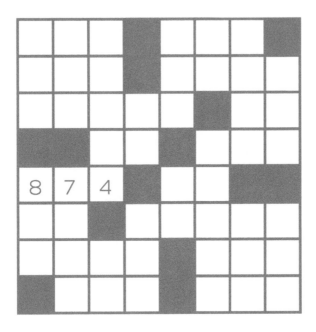

TWO DIGITS	THREE DIGITS	FOUR DIGITS	FIVE DIGITS
23	124	3467	20475
24	192	4320	53813
29	294	5649	54434
34	312	7535	69828
46	345		
74	365		
84	548		
85	592		
	608		
	620		
	735		
	762		
	785		
	825		
	884		

ANSWER ON PAGE 220

NUMBER FILL-IN 5

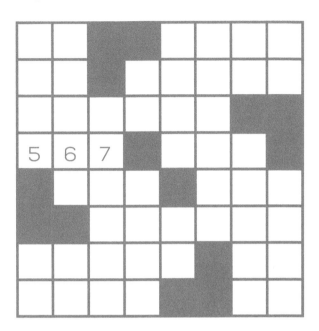

TWO DIGITS

15
23
29
34
35
40
42
50
56
82

THREE DIGITS

202
215
646

FOUR DIGITS

2507
3555
5377
6435
6522
6728

FIVE DIGITS

24121
43570
45792
46462

SIX DIGITS

171450
435514
541024
774065

ANSWER ON PAGE 221

CHALLENGE
LEVEL 2

Sudokus

You will find this group of five sudokus more challenging, as there are fewer numbers already correctly placed in the grid to get you started. As a result, it will be harder to locate those "sure fits" to fill in that move you toward solving the puzzle. But hang in there. Those "sure fits" are there to be found!

SUDOKU 6

		9	6	2	8			
	1		7				5	
				3		9	7	
		6			5	2		7
			9		3			
1		7	2			5		
	6	4		5				
	5				7		2	
			8	1	2	6		

SUDOKU 7

5					3		1	
	3		8	1			2	
		4		6	2			
	1			4		7		6
9		6				1		2
2		5		3			8	
			9	8		2		
	9			5	7		6	
	6		3					9

ANSWER ON PAGE 222

SUDOKU 8

3	5		4	9				1
	4				1			
	1	9	8		5			
8			1				5	2
		5	9		8	7		
1	9				3			6
			5		9	3	8	
			6				7	
9				1	4		6	5

SUDOKU 9

6			9	7				4
9		2		3				
	5		8		6			1
			7			9		
	6						2	
		5			2			
1			5		8		7	
				1		4		9
5				6	7			2

ANSWER ON PAGE 222

SUDOKU 10

		9		6				
	6		7		4	1	5	
5				2		8		6
		6		8	2	4		
	5						8	
		1	3	5		9		
6		5		4				3
	1	4	2		5		9	
				9		5		

ANSWER ON PAGE 223

CHALLENGE
LEVEL 2

Number Searches

For this group of five more challenging number search puzzles, we've increased the grid size a little and added more embedded numbers for you to find. Also, there are only five circled digits (which represent either the first digit of an embedded number or a spot where two embedded numbers intersect) to help you get started.

Your challenge is ramped up even further starting with this group of puzzles, in that the numbers are embedded in the grid in all directions. That is, a number might be embedded so it reads horizontally from left to right, or vertically from top to bottom. That order might also be reversed, so the number reads backward from right to left or from bottom to top. We've also embedded some numbers diagonally, and these can be read either from top to bottom or from bottom to top. But I say the bigger the challenge, the more the fun!

NUMBER SEARCH 6

```
0 2 9 1 4 7 6 0 5 4 6 1
7 1 1 9 3 1 6 5 9 6 9 6
7 5 6 6 8 0 6 5 9 5 2 3
8 7 5 8 0 7 6 9 2 2 1 (1)
0 7 7 5 7 7 2 3 6 0 1 3
6 8 2 4 6 9 5 2 3 8 3 5
7 4 3 5 4 7 3 0 3 1 8 3
8 4 (4) 6 7 5 4 (2) 8 5 1 4
7 5 9 2 8 2 4 4 7 8 (9) 6
0 5 3 7 3 5 9 (6) 2 5 6 6
1 3 2 0 6 3 3 2 4 2 1 0
8 2 2 8 8 3 3 4 5 6 6 8
```

107876	4278	64544777	7605
1353466	4455	66543	883
239786	456765	69537	92113
3042	6005	75325	953227899

ANSWER ON PAGE 223

NUMBER SEARCH 7

```
7  5  6  3  2  7  7  5  3  7  5  4
5  4  8  3  5  6  1  9  6  2  9  3
5  0  5  2  4  2  9  4  4  5  9  8
7  5  1  9  9  4  7  1  5  3  5  6
1  3  9  4  1  7  7  5  2  2  3  5
3  0  6  3  1  0  2  4  0  4  2  6
8  5  8  9  4  1  9  1  2  1  4  7
8  9  2  4  8  7  1  3  9  9  1  9
3  1  4  7  5  1  2  7  4  8  4  2
0  2  9  8  4  4  2  6  3  0  0  2
1  3  0  2  9  9  8  4  7  2  1  0
1  7  8  6  9  4  2  1  2  1  3  4
```

12946	34474	64520294	73577
3002	347267	6942	745910934
31212	5571388	711	7656834
31475	57253	732195	9953241

ANSWER ON PAGE 223

NUMBER SEARCH 8

```
7  8  5  9  7  8  3  4  8  ③  0  4
6  1  9  9  4  6  9  2  2  4  6  3
6  3  5  7  7  7  9  2  9  4  4  7
2  9  1  8  5  8  6  3  3  5  8  9
3  0  0  5  4  3  8  3  9  5  3  9
5  ⓪  2  4  8  8  ②  9  4  6  3  8
1  2  1  4  3  4  0  4  5  1  2  3
5  8  9  9  7  3  3  8  6  1  0  7
8  7  2  9  7  3  1  1  3  6  8  2
4  9  9  1  7  9  3  5  5  6  0  9
6  0  5  0  ①  0  1  4  7  ⑨  5  8
9  5  4  5  4  5  6  1  2  9  9  0
```

1008763	34455611	54545	7948
2009318	3899734	60501	8597410
31599	44892	6623	97532466
3226	4833	771	997423

ANSWER ON PAGE 224

NUMBER SEARCH 9

```
4  3  4  5  9  5  4  0  1  6  2  8
1  6  2  7  8  5  7  9  0  4  1  6
1  2  3  8  7  5  5  7  2  5  9  0
1  9  0  8  7  1  7  9  5  3  2  0
2  4  1  5  2  4  8  0  9  0  5  2
7  2  7  1  8  3  7  8  0  9  9  3
6  5  5  9  2  9  1  3  0  5  2  1
9  7  0  5  2  3  0  9  0  6  9  0
5  2  0  1  2  3  5  7  1  4  9  5
1  4  8  5  6  1  0  2  9  3  1  1
2  4  6  8  3  7  2  4  0  2  5  9
3  0  3  4  2  1  1  3  2  4  4  7
```

1209847	4088	59672111	73041
23465	4273864	645309	757575
3034211	4345954	65841	860023
331	46382319	7259	88177

ANSWER ON PAGE 224

NUMBER SEARCH 10

```
5  2  3 (4) 3  5  3  5  6  9 (2) 5
2  0  3  7  1  8  3  5  0  3  7  8
8  7  9  5  0  3  1  8  9 (6) 4  3
6  7 (4) 8  5  1  6  0  3  8  0  7
5  0  3  6  7  3  3  9  5  6  0  1
4  7  1  8  3  2  8  1  4  7  3  7
3  5  2  0  4  5  0  8  8  1  5  0
2  3  7  3  0  9  6  3  5  1  8  0
1  5  7  5  9  3  8  1  3  3  7  6
9  5  7  0  5  3  2  0  8  1  8  7
5  5  1  4  8  3  7  2  2  4  3  3
3  0 (6) 8  4  9  0  5  0  7  3  1
```

109901	296535	51178	654321
1313	4325	5550	68490507
203	4635618	60071	6867113
239032437	496314	643	943127

ANSWER ON PAGE 224

CHALLENGE
LEVEL 2

Number Fill-Ins

For this set of number fill-ins, we ramped up your challenge by boosting the size of the grids to be filled from 8 × 8 to 11 × 11.

NUMBER FILL-IN 6

TWO DIGITS

32
44
46
55
57
60

THREE DIGITS

101
127
223
227
313
335
386
397
410
445
453
564
637
716
765
777
865
876
901
918

FOUR DIGITS

2343
3256
3897
4813
5565
6258
6477

FIVE DIGITS

47945
49880
51630
99566

SIX DIGITS

449929
453900
643841
948570

SEVEN DIGITS

2591216
3164869
3435605
7482425

EIGHT DIGITS

24596974
48376275

ANSWER ON PAGE 225

NUMBER FILL-IN 7

TWO DIGITS

13
18
41
53
54
73
84
97

THREE DIGITS

101
123
145
232
386
416
431
432
548
563
611
680
745
754
789
792
861
967

			▓				▓			
			▓			▓		▓		
					▓					
▓		9	9	4	5	▓				
	▓							▓	▓	▓
		▓			▓					
▓										
			▓						▓	
					▓					
			▓				▓			
				▓			▓			

FOUR DIGITS

2407
2743
3291
7727
8582
9281
9518
9654
9787

FIVE DIGITS

31150
35210
37073
54631
67549
84578

SIX DIGITS

501668
521900

SEVEN DIGITS

5937414
5974394
6872519
7404438

EIGHT DIGITS

19034467
48573034

ANSWER ON PAGE 225

NUMBER FILL-IN 8

TWO DIGITS

37

39

40

44

45

54

55

61

70

74

77

94

THREE DIGITS

162

177

271

334

391

423

431

473

496

627

731

934

948

986

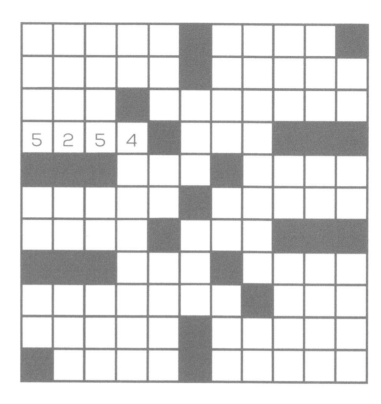

FOUR DIGITS

1934

3318

3443

3475

4105

4142

4366

5695

5960

7120

7480

7543

9985

FIVE DIGITS

25667

30334

35065

38475

42378

46774

54971

61976

SEVEN DIGITS

2318140

5678434

EIGHT DIGITS

40861867

42751872

ANSWER ON PAGE 225

NUMBER FILL-IN 9

TWO DIGITS

33
50

THREE DIGITS

100
143
154
163
223
237
238
243
244
256
263
276
286
305
342
352
365
452
464
554
563
597

641
723
731
733
753
764
806
827
857
923

FOUR DIGITS

5207

FIVE DIGITS

17854
23911
47712
52884
78152
78734
84006
87334

SIX DIGITS

486531
507542

SEVEN DIGITS

6542811
6591933
7203875
7285432

ANSWER ON PAGE 225

NUMBER FILL-IN 10

TWO DIGITS

24

44

THREE DIGITS

234

307

309

329

458

785

809

853

908

FOUR DIGITS

1336

1368

2165

2170

2311

2375

3110

3152

3373

4305

5378

6438

6534

7531

7756

9123

FIVE DIGITS

25739

51386

56878

84539

93467

99283

SIX DIGITS

209836

213852

228212

360534

406335

812635

863508

957254

SEVEN DIGITS

5745602

7634893

8384188

9225342

ANSWER ON PAGE 226

CHALLENGE
LEVEL 3

Sudokus

For this, your most challenging level of sudokus, we've removed even more of the "starter" numbers already positioned on the grid when you begin working on the puzzles. They can be solved, but it will require additional work. Good luck!

SUDOKU 11

			3				9	
1	4	6	9					
9			7		1	8		6
		9			8			
	5	8				7	2	
			5			4		
7		5	2		3			8
					7	6	5	2
	1				5			

SUDOKU 12

		5						
3	4		7	2				5
1	8			3				
6		7		8	4			1
8	2						4	7
5			6	9		8		2
				5			6	3
2				6	3		1	4
						2		

ANSWER ON PAGE 227

SUDOKU 13

8			5			7	1	
		7						
	1			4			9	6
	9	8			5			
	4			7			2	
			1			6	7	
1	2			3			8	
						9		
	8	5			1			3

SUDOKU 14

4					1		6	7
			7	5				
		7			3	8		5
				7	5	9		
		8				7		
		6	8	1				
3		4	5			2		
				4	9			
9	7		6					8

ANSWER ON PAGE 227

SUDOKU 15

		2		8				
		4	3	1				8
8		1		5	7			
3		7	5			1		
	4						9	
		6			2	7		5
			9	2		8		1
2				4	8	9		
				6		4		

ANSWER ON PAGE 228

CHALLENGE
LEVEL 3

Number Searches

For this group of the five hardest number search puzzles, we've increased the amount of numbers to be found and enlarged the grid. Additionally, there are only four circled digits in each puzzle (each of which is placed in a spot where two embedded numbers intersect). Have fun uncovering the hidden numbers!

NUMBER SEARCH 11

```
3  4  5  8  5  6  3  7  8  1  1  9  0
3  4  3  1  8  9  0  3  0  7  5  4  6
2  9  4  7  8  3  8  0  9  8  3  5  3
2  1  4  5  1  9  2  3  8  9  0  1  4
2  1  2  0  4  5  9  1  2  4  5  6  8
7  4  3  7  0  6  0  8  3  7  1  5  5
9  3  1  8  9  8  7  4  1  0  6  1  0
3  9  8  2  9  4  5  9  2  7  0  6  9
9  8  5  3  8  3  7  0  5  1  4  9  2
0  3  4  8  9  0  5  9  3  2  9  8  9
8  4  3  0  4  2  1  0  3  8  6  5  2
4  0  7  8  0  7  2  7  2  7  2  7  3
1  8  7  7  3  2  5  4  1  7  6  6  8
```

17668	22279	458563781	7272727
1877325	389471	516516	7546
19576	423185	544	893411
20520	4371504	63485092	
213009	444398	679526	

ANSWER ON PAGE 228

NUMBER SEARCH 12

```
3  3  9  7  2  5  8  3  1  3  4  5  6
1  2 (3) 5  0  9  4  6  9  8  4 (3) 6
8  4  0  5  2  4  1  8  5  0  8  4  2
0  3  1  6  7  3  9  2  2  4  0  5  4
5  8  4  1  2  8  6  7  2  2  5  7  7
(5) 3  8  9  6  2  7  1  3  3  0  1  2
6  7  2  4  7  6  9  0  8  4  2  8  4
5  1  0  2  6  7  4  2  6  0  5  8  7
9  9  6  3  2  4  1  2  9  5  4  5  9
0  2  3  2  6  0  9  8  7  5  1  2  1
9  0  5  1  3 (8) 1  5  0  0  4  7  9
4  3  7  6  4  7  4  3  3  8  7  2  1
5  9  8  5  4  9  1  0  5  6  2  8  9
```

1411	36840	54892	91919
302917	38421972	56590945	973455
33972583	50047	6543	
34571	526272	742742	
357870651	5389	89649053	

ANSWER ON PAGE 228

NUMBER SEARCH 13

```
2  3  4  8  9  5  8  7  5  4  6  8  4
2  4  9  6  0  9  0  6  3  8  1  9  4
4  1  7  7  7  1  0  7  0  3  2  9  3
5  8  6  0  9  5  4  8  6  5  1  6  2
6  5  7  9  9  6  7  3  5  8  2  4  9
8  7  1  0  8  9  2  2  3  9  1  5  1
6  6  8  5  9  0  1  2  9  5  2  6  7
9  8  7  3  0  2  5  4  8  0  3  2  5
7  5  2  4  6  9  3  8  9  3  1  7  8
4  6  7  8  9  7  6  5  0  7  6  3  2
3  2  6  8  2  1  0  9  6  4  5  5  7
2  6  2  9  9  6  7  3  6  0  2  7  1
2  6  1  2  3  0  4  8  8  9  8  6  5
```

121212	24960	5799	8403
17771	3200472	686542	96969
192734	358950	7192344	
2348958754	437468575	74322	
235608	57290137	757	

ANSWER ON PAGE 229

NUMBER SEARCH 14

```
4 1 6 2 2 4 8 9 3 5 8 9 (5)
4 5 7 7 6 8 1 2 5 7 6 4 3
7 1 8 (4) 5 6 7 2 9 1 8 2 5
6 5 9 6 7 1 8 4 1 9 2 5 8
6 7 8 5 1 3 3 8 3 7 6 5 9
4 2 6 5 6 7 8 1 1 8 7 6 6
3 5 0 4 0 8 7 1 9 7 5 6 (3)
2 4 3 0 1 4 3 1 5 2 1 5 8
3 9 6 3 6 0 1 3 1 8 3 4 6
2 0 4 4 6 7 6 4 2 1 1 2 4
3 7 9 0 5 3 0 4 3 8 4 7 2
1 5 7 3 2 8 9 3 2 8 5 6 3
2 3 7 7 1 2 2 3 3 (7) 6 9 8
```

17732	369853	4567291	907
248935895	40511	4738158	97563
336393	421124	5489317464	9876
33865	437006	64106427	
35711	447664323	89673	

ANSWER ON PAGE 229

NUMBER SEARCH 15

```
2  5  7  8  7  8  7  8  4 (1) 6  8  7
6 (8) 7  4  8  0  4  6  3  7  8  0  1
2  9  4  3  2  8  7  5  2  3  6  6  4
5  2  1  5  4  5  8  0  4  1  5  9  2
3  3  0  1  9  3  5  4  3  6  5  7  8
7  0  1  5  6  0  3  0  2  1  4  7  6
6  7  0  6  8  5  7  5  0  2  4  9  4
5  6  9  7  2  3  8  0  1  3  4  1  0
4  0  3  7  6  8  9  7  4 (6) 3  4  9
5  8  7  4  0  3  6  4  8  7  9  5  9
2  1  7  3  2  6  8  4  3  5  2  4  1
1  4  8  7  6  3  7  3  0  4  0  9  3
(5) 8  3  3  2  3  8  7  9  2  2  2  4
```

101093	332	516943	878787
1307364745	35277	5524	90403
1687	37486496	589230	9904
25376545215	46632	638531	
284590	5100932	792224	

ANSWER ON PAGE 229

CHALLENGE
LEVEL 3

Number Fill-Ins

To make this last set of five number fill-ins more challenging, the size of the grid has been increased once again to 13 × 13. That means more numbers to juggle, but more fun, too!

NUMBER FILL-IN 11

THREE DIGITS

100	
116	
194	
213	
218	
238	
251	
276	
284	
321	
345	
358	
374	
411	
428	
432	
461	
468	
533	
546	
581	
595	
698	
775	
833	
872	
892	
956	

FOUR DIGITS		FIVE DIGITS
1290	5774	10938
1852	5842	21548
2038	6287	36449
3040	6468	51605
3210	6533	
3565	7399	
3723	7814	
4676	7953	
4857	8766	
5742	8772	
	9823	

CONTINUED

SEVEN DIGITS	EIGHT DIGITS	NINE DIGITS
3541185	22392694	452495660
3834025	22805426	452945858
4833298	54937856	
5321156	75431767	

ANSWER ON PAGE 230

NUMBER FILL-IN 12

TWO DIGITS

14
28
31
59

THREE DIGITS

103
107
318
376
405
411
423
441
459
528
634
653
698
864
886
930

FOUR DIGITS

1466
2009
2356
2385
3005
3413
3727
4544
4894
5306
5437
5967
6454
6582
6590
6765
6857
7332
8529
8654
9584

FIVE DIGITS

13785
18378
34278
39844
43147
43433
47432
48168

CONTINUED

48369
49561
54371
55758
64265
86743

SIX DIGITS

128654
348569
351548
594803
760462
899368

SEVEN DIGITS

8062573
8475853
8734864
8769301

ANSWER ON PAGE 230

NUMBER FILL-IN 13

TWO DIGITS

42

56

64

98

THREE DIGITS

100

107

114

178

245

338

341

342

345

353

356

394

395

420

423

432

450

456

488

490

547

556

581

636

658

698

794

837

875

943

958

FOUR DIGITS

2663

3447

3488

4335

4483

4714

4909

4956

5041

5489

5528

5566

5655

7321

8209

8474

9114

9358

CONTINUED

LEVEL 3

FIVE DIGITS

12385

24169

30135

68753

75436

75968

86436

93820

SIX DIGITS

151876

326553

564828

859190

SEVEN DIGITS

3564312

3575483

EIGHT DIGITS

64446343

85758400

ANSWER ON PAGE 230

NUMBER FILL-IN 14

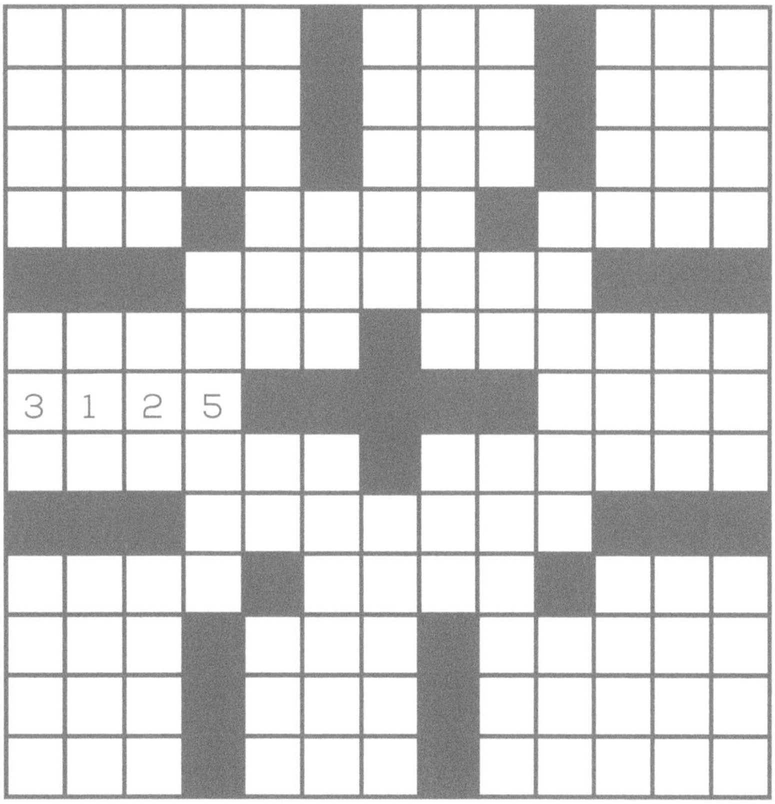

TWO DIGITS

78
88

THREE DIGITS

123
216
236
237
246
310
327
346
378
446
463
475
556
561
564
568
608
638
678
723
753
785
907
939
944
955

FOUR DIGITS

2624
3225
3746
4833
4851
5419
5548
5963
5978
6637
6662
6878
7823
8374
9086
9420
9446

FIVE DIGITS

22678
23676
24581
24831
26468
39469
60566
74247

CONTINUED

SIX DIGITS

120883

206272

245743

325754

387249

459854

737852

903784

911594

937445

SEVEN DIGITS

2956873

4856702

ANSWER ON PAGE 230

NUMBER FILL-IN 15

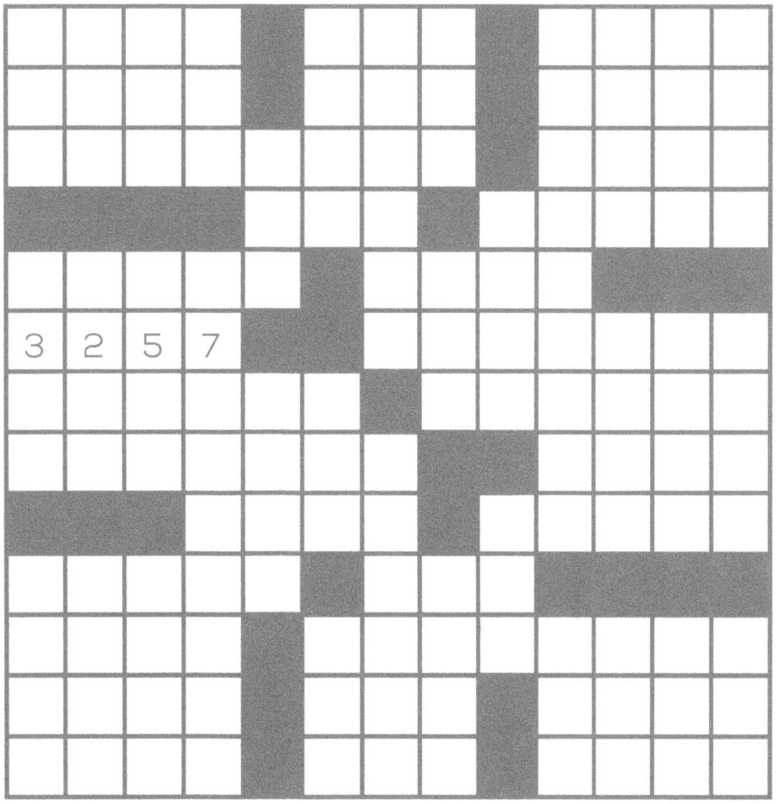

THREE DIGITS

129
164
195
209
249
254
295
324
352
418
419
421
508
548
572
599
818
825
884
984

FOUR DIGITS

1328
1454
1587
2126
2260
2346
2347
2351
2416
2472
2552
2751
3232
3298
3558
3652
4328
4448
4894
4996
5003
5198
5304
6834
7169
7276
7337
8610
9803

FIVE DIGITS

12148
15789
39516
48210

SIX DIGITS

268923
364796
404931
961341

SEVEN DIGITS

1094747
8076453

EIGHT DIGITS

47452458
48258544

NINE DIGITS

472884125
479621437

ANSWER ON PAGE 231

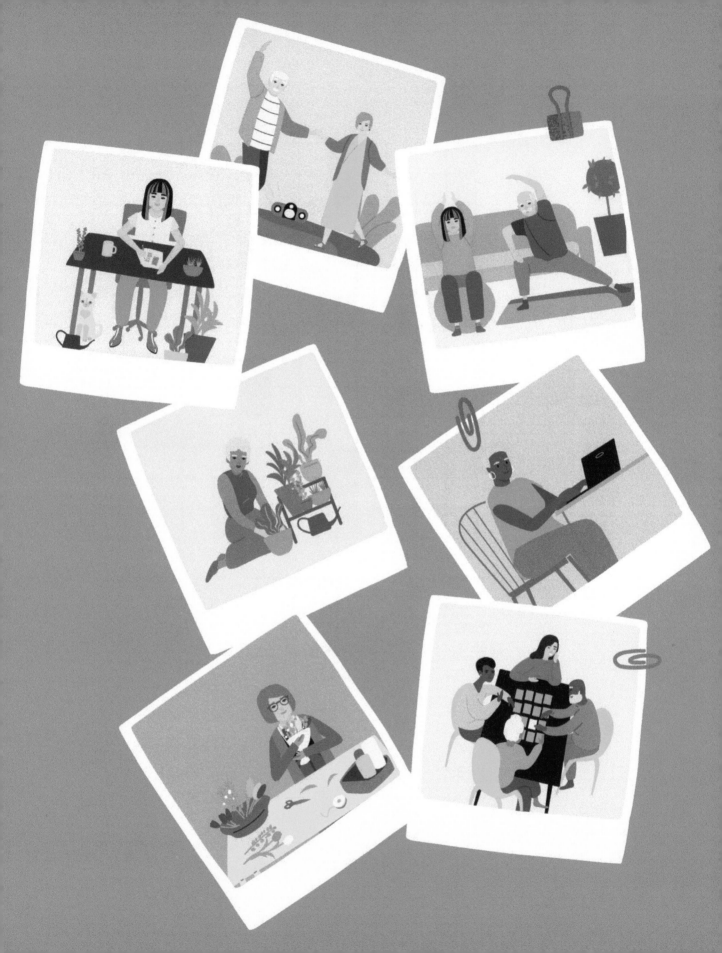

CHAPTER 4

Let's Do This! 30 Engaging Activity Tips

As helpful as routines are, sometimes we need to shake things up. Our bodies and minds love to keep things as simple as possible, which often means shifting to simpler and simpler tasks. I'm a fan of simplicity, but not when it means the limits of our abilities go unchecked for long periods of time. By monitoring our accuracy and progress on less familiar activities, we can push those limits, challenging our brain to adapt.

Though creating opportunities that require our minds to think twice can feel uncomfortable and even frustrating at times, it keeps us sharper for longer. These opportunities can be both mental and physical. As described earlier, procedural memory can involve our body recalling how to sequence movements almost automatically or with very few cues. With practice, such steps become easier, such as in Beanbag Bocce (page 178).

And since our mood can affect how efficiently we think, engaging in mood-boosting activities can facilitate thinking. This is shown in activities such as Gratitude Express (page 140) and International Tea Time (page 142). Engaging in such uplifting, kinesthetic, or critical-thinking activities demands more responsiveness from your brain, resulting in more densely connected brain cells. Now that you know the mind processes involved, it's time to take action with these 30 step-by-step activity ideas.

Finally, although most of these activities can be done anywhere, some do take place in parks, cafés, or your neighborhood sidewalks. If someone normally accompanies you when you venture out, make sure they are in on the plans.

Gratitude Express

Do you remember that feeling—before bills with your name on them existed—of reaching into the mailbox and pulling out a postcard addressed to you? Someone thought of you and went to the trouble of picking out a card, writing a note just for you, and sending it off to find its way to your spot on the map.

You can re-create that feeling now for someone in your life. Although the Pony Express took 10 days to make deliveries about 2,000 miles away, now we can have handmade cards delivered via the Gratitude Express in just two or three days, coast to coast.

Writing letters is also good for the soul. Research shows that you can increase your happiness and life satisfaction while decreasing depressive symptoms simply by writing a note of gratitude to someone in your life.

NECESSITIES:

Card stock (postcard-style also works)

Colored pens

Stamps

Optional: stickers, photos, glue stick/Mod Podge

1. Think of someone you are thankful for or who inspires gratitude in you.

2. Locate their address.

3. Pull out the card stock and mark up one side with any designs, stickers, stamps, and photos. It can be as crafty or as simple as you'd like. Just draw a little star, a heart, or other doodle in the middle of the page for a very basic, yet still personalized, card. The most important part is your message on the other side!

4. Flip over the postcard and mark a line down the middle. Write the recipient's address on the right side.

5. Now it's time to express your gratitude for an act of kindness someone did for you, whether brightening your day with a phone call or a compliment, offering support during a rough time, or just being a person you can count on no matter what. If you find it hard to get the right words out the first time, draft your note on another piece of paper first, then write it out on the postcard. This limits do-overs and scratch-outs from appearing on your final card.

6. Your message can be simple and sweet or verbose. The important thing is that you share your sentiment with your recipient.

7. Add a postage stamp and mail to your intended recipient.

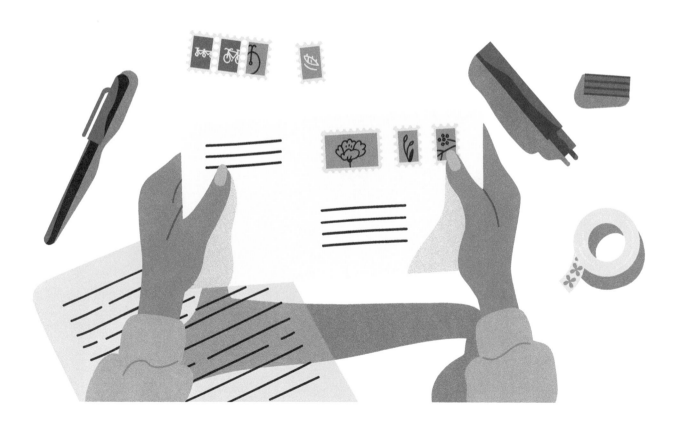

International Tea Time

Tea has been enjoyed for thousands of years, and the practice of drinking tea is elevated to an art form in many cultures. From East Indian spicy chai to ceremonial matcha tea, the variety of teas is immense. The visuals of swirling steam or clouds of milk in tea are mesmerizing, and the aroma can be intoxicating and mentally stimulating.

Many tea varieties contain caffeine or bioactive compounds that have brain benefits, such as improved mood or memory, and antioxidant effects. This activity includes a number of tea experiences for you to explore. Be sure to note which ones you especially enjoy, so you can re-create the experience in the future.

If you don't need the extra energy (aka caffeine), skip it, and buy one of the many decaffeinated varieties available in grocery stores, online, and in tea houses and specialty tea shops. Join up with a friend or have tea time solo!

NECESSITIES:

Tea (see following list for types and accompaniments)

Hot water

Cup

Straining device (mesh, tea strainer, teapot, etc.)

The following list of tea styles begins with the simplest setup and continues on to more involved tea processes.

Green: This delicate, bright-flavored tea from China comes in many varieties.

1. One trick to making green tea is having the right water temperature (~170 degrees Fahrenheit). If you don't have a thermometer, stop heating the water just before it boils.

2. Place the green tea bag and water into a cup, and steep for 1 minute.

3. Remove the bag and serve.

> Moroccan Mint: A customary sign of hospitality in Morocco, this sweet, mint green tea is typically made with loose gunpowder green tea leaves, but you can use what's on hand.

1. Mix 2 cups boiling water with two green tea bags (or 2 teaspoons of loose tea).

2. Steep for 2 minutes, then remove tea bags/strain out tea leaves.

3. Stir in sugar until delightfully sweet and add sprigs of spearmint. Sip on this aromatic treat!

> Chai: An East Indian delight, this creamy, aromatic tea warms the senses and the heart. "Chai" actually means "tea," so, chai tea (as Westerners say) is the equivalent of saying "tea tea." A more accurate title is "masala chai," meaning "spiced tea."

1. Gather a few tablespoons of masala (buy it from a market or combine ginger, cloves, fennel, cardamom, cinnamon, and/or star anise).

2. Simmer the spices in 1 cup of milk and 1 cup of water for 5 minutes or so.

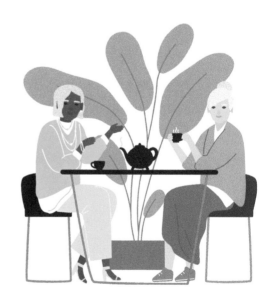

3. Drop in 2 to 3 black tea bags or teaspoons of loose black tea. Turn off heat, cover, and let steep for about 4 minutes.

4. Strain and serve.

Smoothie Time

A smoothie is a fantastic treat that's good for the brain and the body. Packed with fruits and veggies (yes, veggies too!), it offers a nutritient-rich and easy meal or beverage. It also can include brain-healthy fatty acids (found in flaxseed, chia seeds, and avocado) and slow-burning fuels (like protein found in nuts and nut butters) that facilitate a clear mind.

A smoothie is a colorful way to brighten your morning and is an easy on-the-go food if you have to head out the door quickly. Make a smoothie out of the mix-and-match lists on page 145. Some combinations are hearty and decadent, while others are bright and refreshing. Track your favorites on a piece of paper or in a notebook for future reference.

Smoothies are a carefree way to explore in the kitchen. It might get a little noisy, but the results are worth it. Though they don't keep particularly well, they refresh pretty easily with a zip in the blender. Make yours ahead of time, or drink it down right away!

NECESSITIES:

Items from at least the first two lists on page 145
Blender

---

1. Pick the ingredients that suit your mood. Rich and hearty? Stick to the bottom end of the lists. Light and refreshing? Stay toward the top.

2. Look over the lists of bases, fruits, extras, and accents. Purchase the ingredients you would like to try from the lists, or use what you have on hand.

3. Place a handful of each of the first three ingredients in the blender, then add a dash or more of the accent. Hint: Start with less. You can always add more to your taste later.

4. For a cold smoothie, drop in ice cubes before you blend, or freeze some ingredients.

5. If you don't like cold smoothies, microwave frozen ingredients a bit before blending, or add some hot water to the blender.

6. Sip and enjoy!

BASE	MAIN	SECONDARY	ACCENT
Water	Watermelon	Açai	Lime juice
Lemonade	Blueberries	Spinach	Mint leaves
Apple juice	Strawberries	Mango	Ginger (dry or fresh)
Orange juice	Raspberries	Sweet potato (cooked)	Cinnamon (powdered)
Milk	Peaches	Yogurt	Chia seeds
Rice milk	Banana	Cottage cheese	Peanut/almond butter
Almond milk			Cocoa powder
Coconut milk			Protein powder

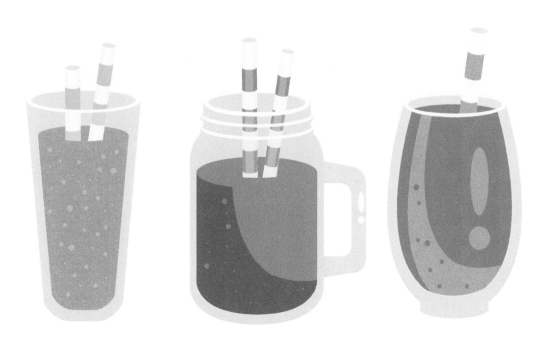

Mindful Eating

Have you ever found yourself at the end of a meal wondering, "How am I already finished eating?" If so, your attention likely wandered during the dining experience. Maybe you were distracted by the events of your day or engaged in wonderful conversation with a dining companion.

This activity will remind you that paying attention to each bite of a delicious meal—whether a four-course tasting menu or a peanut butter and jelly sandwich—deepens your experience. This draws on the practice of mindfulness, which means bringing your attention to the present moment, on purpose and nonjudgmentally. You might even find that you feel more satisfied at the end of a mindful meal. Mindfulness cultivates both cognitive and emotional abilities, including developing greater resilience to stress, and best of all, it can be done in just a few steps, with only your mind as a guide.

NECESSITIES:

Any food (such as grapes, a single chocolate chip, a smoothie, or a full meal)

A quiet place (optional, but preferred)

1. Pick your food, whether it's raisins, a power bar, or a full meal.

2. Find a quiet place to eat.

3. Using your eyes only—no eating yet!—observe your food's texture for at least 20 seconds. Is it rough or smooth? Are the edges even or crooked? If your attention wanders, gently bring it back to the texture of your food.

4. Using your hands or a fork, examine the substance of your food. Is it firm or soft? How does it move when pushed? Do this for at least 20 seconds.

5. Breathe in the aroma of your food. Notice its fragrance or absence of fragrance. Notice if its scent lingers or if it only lasts for a few seconds. Notice any reactions of your body to this food. Do you start salivating or have a reaction to sweet or sour smells? Do this for at least 20 seconds.

6. Place a bite-sized portion of the food in your mouth. Notice the reaction of your body and your senses. Pay attention to the shape of the food as you chew it and the sensation of swallowing it.

7. Before your next bite, notice the lingering flavor or texture in your mouth. Notice if your instinct is to take another bite or if you are present with the flavor. Allow your attention to stay with the sensations in your mouth for at least 20 seconds.

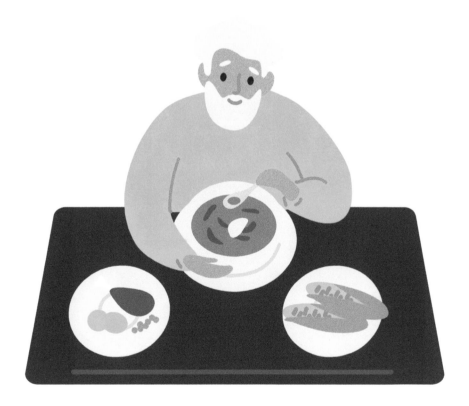

Breathing Practice

You may think you've been breathing for long enough to know how it's done, but believe it or not, we can all use practice with this life-sustaining function. There are a few breathing tips you may not have learned just yet.

Our breath is linked to our sense of safety, calm, and relaxation, so we can use it to switch gears emotionally. For example, if you want to slow your heart rate or reduce irritation, take some deep breaths into your belly. Full-belly breathing stimulates the vagus nerve, which runs just behind your lungs and diaphragm in your upper belly. This nerve tells your brain that "all is well," prompting your brain to tell your body to relax. You can also harness your attention with your breath, making it a great exercise to increase your ability to focus.

This exercise can be done anywhere at nearly any time. It can be most useful to engage in it regularly, so your body gets in the habit of tuning into your breath for self-relaxation. Whether you're feeling stressed or just want to continue through your day with ease, directing your attention to your breathing will foster greater inner peace.

NECESSITIES:

A quiet place

Consider having someone read the following steps aloud to you while you follow along, so you can focus entirely on your breathing. You also have the option to listen to recorded audio online (DoctorOlson.com/media). You may also read the steps out loud while recording yourself on your smartphone, then play it back when you are ready to do the exercise.

---

1. Sit or lie comfortably in a quiet space.

2. Begin by relaxing your face.

3. Place a hand on your stomach and a hand on your chest, just over your sternum.

4. Breathe naturally and notice if your chest is rising more than your stomach. One goal is to expand the stomach with each inhale, while allowing your chest to remain relatively still. It will move a little.

5. On your next inhale, inhale deeply and fully. Feel your belly expand, while your chest stays relatively still. Hold the breath for a couple seconds, then slowly exhale. Notice your belly falling back in.

6. Continue with this process of a slow, full inhale, a brief hold at the top, then a long, slow exhale.

7. If your mind wanders, bring it back to the rise and fall of your belly or to the air moving in and out of your lungs.

8. Continue for as long as you'd like, perhaps starting with just a few minutes at a time.

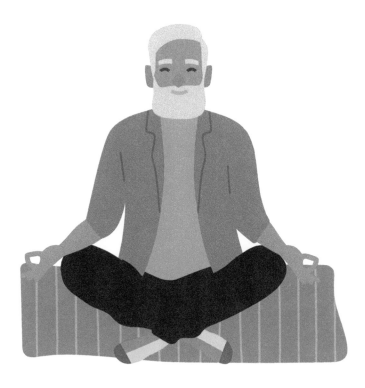

Cloud Finder

Cloudy days aren't all bad. Sometimes they offer the opportunity to explore with science and our imaginations. Plus, studies show that time in nature can boost mood and thinking abilities. Clouds—essentially suspended collections of water—form different shapes depending on the direction and force of the air, atmospheric pressure, and cold and warm weather fronts. Bring the following cloud key outdoors, along with a chair or blanket, and gaze up to the sky. What do you see?

Identifying clouds, which come in many shapes and sizes, is a good mental exercise. For an extra bit of imagination and creativity, maybe you'd like to point out any shapes or characters you see in the clouds, once you identify what kind they are.

NECESSITIES:

Cloud key

A view of at least a partially cloudy sky

Optional: blanket or chair

See if you can identify the cloud types that are present in the sky above you:

- **Altocumulus:** These mid-level, grayish-white groups of clouds—with one part darker than the other—may indicate thunderstorms if it's a warm and humid morning.

- **Altostratus:** These mid-level gray clouds with lots of sky coverage cause the sun to appear watery or hazy. These clouds harken an extended rain or snow storm.

- **Cirrocumulus:** These small, rounded puffs often appear in long rows high in the sky and are usually white but sometimes gray. When several cirrocumulus clouds are present, it's called a "mackerel sky" because it looks like fish scales. You'll see them in winter, indicating fair yet cold weather.

- **Cirrus:** These long, fine, white streaks are high in the sky. Also called "mare's tails," because they're shaped like the tail of a horse, cirrus clouds often coincide with fair weather.

- **Cumulonimbus:** These clouds grow vertically up to 10 kilometers high, where winds flatten their tops. Known as thunderstorm clouds, they can produce heavy rain, hail, lightning, and even tornadoes.

- **Cumulus:** Puffy, like cottonballs, these clouds suspend lower in the sky and often have a flat bottom.

- **Nimbostratus:** These dark gray clouds appear low in the sky and often coincide with persistent rain or snow.

- **Stratocumulus:** These low, lumpy, gray clouds resemble a thick and loose wire mesh and often produce a light rain.

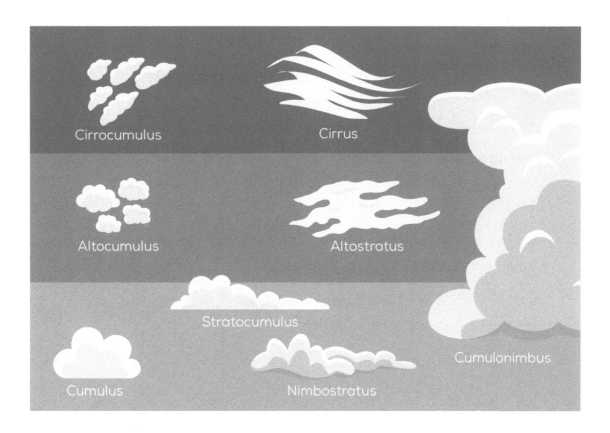

Balloon Ball

Socializing doesn't always need to involve talking. You can learn a lot about a person by how they play ball, and in this case, it's balloon ball.

Not all climates, spaces, or human bodies are conducive to running around and chasing after balls, so the slowness and gentleness of balloons are helpful. They offer a challenge in coordination without much risk to your body or your furniture, since this game is played indoors. It can also be played in your backyard on a day that is not windy. The added challenge of tracking the score mentally, plus other modifications, makes this a stimulating, multifaceted activity for the mind and the body.

This can be a tricky game to learn, however. Hitting a balloon may feel a little wonky at first, but once you get the hang of it, it's a fun, social, and portable activity. Get ready to flex your patience, trivia knowledge, and sportsmanship. Gather one or more friends and see whose aim takes the gold!

NECESSITIES:
Standard balloons (at least a few, just in case a couple pop)
Rope, towels, or other item to mark "net line"
Two or more people

1. Blow up a few balloons to their full size. For added challenge, deflate them a bit, which makes the balloons travel less far and sink faster than if they were fully inflated.

2. Designate a space for your "court." This could be the dining table, the living room floor, the backyard, the garage, etc.

3. Designate a "net line" by placing a rope, a few towels, or some other demarcation across the middle of the court.

4. Form evenly numbered teams.

5. One team serves and the other team tries to hit the balloon back across the "net line."

6. Play continues until the balloon lands—gaining a point for the team who hit it across the line last.

7. On each serve, the serving team must state the score of both teams or risk losing their serve.

8. If you'd like to play more cooperatively, ditch the net and teams and try to set a group record for number of hits in a row before the balloon touches the ground.

9. For more brain stimulation, have players sound off U.S. states or presidents (or another category with limited items) whenever they hit the balloon. The first one without an answer when they hit the ball resets the game.

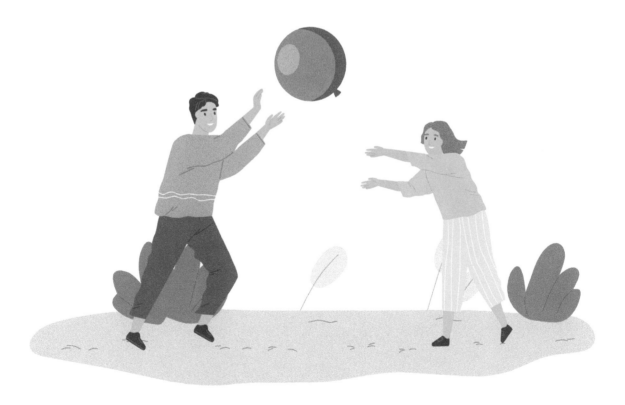

Musical Memories

Music is known to bring back some of our most vivid memories, so let's revisit your favorite decades through their top 10 musical hits. Each song probably won't be your favorite, but it may at least get a laugh or groan out of you.

The following table lists popular songs from the 1950s through the 1990s. Turn on the tunes and sing along—you might be surprised at how many lyrics you remember! Each song listed spent one of the longest times at the top of the charts for the year noted.

You can't help but dance to some of these songs. If it moves you, dance a little and maybe even invite someone to shimmy with you.

NECESSITIES:

Audio system (e.g., smartphone, computer with speakers, MP3 player)

Internet access to retrieve songs from places such as YouTube or Spotify

YEAR	ARTIST	SONG
1950	Anton Karas	*"The Third Man* Theme"
1951	Johnnie Ray and The Four Lads	"Cry"
1952	Kay Starr	"Wheel of Fortune"
1953	Les Paul and Mary Ford	"Vaya con Dios (May God Be with You)"
1954	Kitty Kallen	"Little Things Mean a Lot"
1955	Pérez Prado	"Cherry Pink and Apple Blossom White"
1956	Elvis Presley	"Don't Be Cruel"/"Hound Dog"
1957	Elvis Presley	"All Shook Up"
1958	Domenico Modugno	"Volare (Nel blu dipinto di blu)"

YEAR	ARTIST	SONG
1959	Johnny Horton	"The Battle of New Orleans"
1960	Percy Faith	"Theme from *A Summer Place*"
1961	Bobby Lewis	"Tossin' and Turnin'"
1962	Ray Charles	"I Can't Stop Loving You"
1963	Jimmy Gilmer and the Fireballs	"Sugar Shack"
1964	The Beatles	"I Want to Hold Your Hand"
1965	The Rolling Stones	"(I Can't Get No) Satisfaction"
1966	The Monkees	"I'm a Believer"
1967	Lulu	"To Sir with Love"
1968	The Beatles	"Hey Jude"
1969	Zager and Evans	"In the Year 2525"
1970	The 5th Dimension	"Aquarius/Let the Sunshine In"
1971	Three Dog Night	"Joy to the World"
1972	Looking Glass	"Brandy (You're a Fine Girl)"
1973	Roberta Flack	"Killing Me Softly with His Song"
1974	Barbra Streisand	"The Way We Were"
1975	Captain & Tennille	"Love Will Keep Us Together"
1976	Wings	"Silly Love Songs"
1977	Debby Boone	"You Light Up My Life"
1978	Bee Gees	"Night Fever"
1979	The Knack	"My Sharona"
1980	Blondie	"Call Me"
1981	Diana Ross and Lionel Richie	"Endless Love"

YEAR	ARTIST	SONG
1982	Paul McCartney and Stevie Wonder	"Ebony and Ivory"
1983	The Police	"Every Breath You Take"
1984	Madonna	"Like a Virgin"
1985	Lionel Richie	"Say You, Say Me"
1986	Dionne Warwick	"That's What Friends Are For"
1987	Bon Jovi	"Livin' on a Prayer"
1988	George Michael	"Faith"
1989	Janet Jackson	"Miss You Much"
1990	Sinéad O'Connor	"Nothing Compares 2 U"
1991	Bryan Adams	"(Everything I Do) I Do It for You"
1992	Boyz II Men	"End of the Road"
1993	Whitney Houston	"I Will Always Love You"
1994	Boyz II Men	"I'll Make Love to You"
1995	Mariah Carey and Boyz II Men	"One Sweet Day"
1996	Los Del Rio	"Macarena (Bayside Boys Mix)"
1997	Elton John	"Candle in the Wind"
1998	Brandy and Monica	"The Boy Is Mine"
1999	Santana ft. Rob Thomas	"Smooth"
2000	Santana ft. The Product G&B	"Maria Maria"

New Language Challenge

Language development begins in some of our earliest moments as infants. Over time, our brains are wired to be more attuned to our native language, making foreign languages more difficult to learn as we age. The good news is that introducing a new language is great stimulation for our brain as it works to tune in to new language patterns. In fact, life-long bilingualism is associated with delays in cognitive decline.

Though you might not be up for learning an entire new language, you can try learning a few frequently used phrases—think "hello" or "how are you?"—in one or more new languages. Using unfamiliar languages requires us to use our mouths and voices in ways we typically don't. It also requires that we represent words differently in our minds as their sounds shift.

On the next two pages is a pronunciation guide for a handful of common and fun phrases to use in several languages. You can weave them into conversation with others, or practice on your own as you go about your day. You might not master a new language, but practicing can be a nice brain challenge. Having some basic phrases in your back pocket might also help if you encounter a person who speaks this language, allowing you to form an initial connection.

Don't be afraid to stumble over your words along the way. This is a new skill that requires practice from the very beginning. Just know you're connecting your own brain cells to other cultures by giving it a try!

NECESSITIES:

Foreign translations of common phrases (page 158)
Optional: language-learning book, website, tape, or smartphone app

---

Try the following phrases. Practice them alone or with a partner, and try using them in everyday situations where appropriate—with a Spanish-speaking friend or store owner, for example. If you find it's a fit and enjoy using these phrases in everyday life, you might look into other language-learning resources that could expand upon this introduction, such as Duolingo or Rosetta Stone.

ENGLISH	SPANISH	ITALIAN
Hello!	*¡Hola!* *OH-la*	*Ciao!* *chi-OW*
How are you?	*¿Cómo està?* *Co-moe eh-STAH*	*Come stai?* *Co-may stye?*
I am well.	*Estoy bien.* *Eh-stoy bee-en*	*Sto bene.* *Sto beh-neh*
Thank you.	*Gracias.* *GRAW-see-us*	*Grazie.* *GRAWT-zee-eh*
Excuse me.	*Perdona.* *Pear-DOH-nuh*	*Mi scusi.* *Me SKOO-zee*
Good morning.	*Buenas dias.* *Bwe-NAHS DEE-ahs*	*Buongiorno.* *Boo-ON-gee-OR-no*
Goodnight/ good evening.	*Buenas noches.* *Bwe-NAHS NOH-chess*	*Buonna notte.* *Boo-ON-ah NOH-tay*
My name is (fill in your name).	*Me llamo _____.* *May YAW-moe _____*	*Mi chiamo _____.* *Me key-AM-o _____*
I love you.	*Te quiero.* *Tay key-air-o*	*Ti amo.* *Tee AH-moh*
Happy birthday!	*¡Feliz cumpleaños!* *Feh-LEASE koom-play-on-yose*	*Buon cumpleanno!* *Boo-ON comb-play-on-no*

CHINESE (PHONETICS ONLY)	FARSI
	Salam!
Nee hao	Sah-LOM
	Halet chetore?
Nee hao mah?	Haleh chetoreh?
	Man khubam.
Wuh hen hao	(kh = gentle clearing of the throat)
	Mersi.
Sshyeah-sshyeah	Mer-see
	Bebakhshid.
Dway-boo-chee	BEH-bakh-SHEED
	Sobh bekheir.
Tzao-ahn	Sobh beh-hehr
	Shab bekheir.
Wahn-ahn	Shab beh-hehr
	Esme man _____.
Whoa-de MING-tze-sheh _____.	Es-meh man _____.
	Dúset dáram.
Whoa-EYE-knee	Doo-set dah-ram
	Tavalodet mobarak!
Sheng-reh kwhy-luh	Ta-va-load-et moh-bah-rack

Book Explorers

Reading expands our minds. From the time we first discover stories and facts in books during childhood, our brains actually rewire to accommodate and assimilate new and unique information. Reading and taking in new knowledge results in a more densely constructed network of neurons, or brain cells. Relating facts, solving a mystery story, or following an intriguing plot all fire these neurons.

Let's travel into books right now, just like we did when our reading abilities first blossomed. Rediscovering the joy of exploring books and new ideas offers us endless mind-expanding experiences. Try a genre you've never read before, or pick up a graphic novel or an audiobook. Each story—from nature and history, to memoir and mystery—offers a unique experience.

NECESSITIES:
Books

---

1. Take a trip to the library or a bookstore, or scan through your personal bookshelf section by section. (You might even reorganize your home library while you're at it!)

2. If you have vision challenges or you're simply "not a reader," consider audiobooks or podcasts as an alternative means of accessing stories and information compiled by authors on myriad topics.

3. Jot down any notes, quotes, or book favorites you discover during your excursion. Here are some ideas on topics worth seeking out:

   - **Travel and Leisure:** What are the other people with you on this planet up to? Explore travel guides for an intro or a refresher on the activities and lifestyles of your neighbors near and far.

- **Comic Books and Graphic Novels:** You're likely familiar with comic books, but graphic novels have matured immensely in recent decades, as artists and storytellers render science and history into lively graphic sequences.

- **Cookbooks:** This section makes for great "window shopping." The photos that accompany various recipes can pique your curiosity and have you salivating with anticipation. If you bring a cookbook home, your attempt at a recipe might not match the photo, but it'll be fun trying—and making new dishes is a mentally engaging use of your time!

- **Biography:** If you're looking for some inspiration, the biography section is the spot for discovering lives lived well or in infamy. From poets to politicians, you'll become acquainted with the story of another's life journey.

- **History:** There is a lot of it. Many history books offer fascinating views into the building blocks of civilization, from the earliest humans to the latest fashion craze. Drop in on any century to learn more.

- **Other Sections:** If you're organizing your bookshelves, consider additional categories: fiction (further broken down into romance, mystery, literary, fantasy, and science fiction genres, among others), poetry, humor, photography, art, and do-it-yourself books.

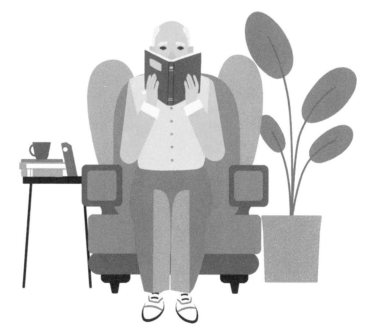

Memory Jar

Each day has highs and lows, but there is generally always something positive to highlight, no matter how small. It might be a good meal, a talk with a friend, or sitting in the sunshine and feeling its warmth on your face. It can be harder to remember those good moments on some days, particularly when mood colors our recollection or steers us to less-uplifting memories. Storing those memories up to return to later can help lift our spirits when it doesn't happen on its own.

Each day or so, write a note about one experience you had that was pleasant, soothing, inspiring, fun, or funny. Tuck this note into your memory jar, and on the days when it feels hard to remember those good moments, pick a few out and relive the positive experiences all over again.

NECESSITIES:

Jar or box

Paper

Pen

1. Locate a jar or a box. Try to find a container the size of a pasta sauce jar or larger, big enough so you don't run out of space for good memories.

2. Pick your paper. Use a small notepad or cut printer paper into large strips. Try using something that will easily fold up and not take up too much room. Use colorful paper for some added pizzazz.

3. Pick a regular time to write. It can be hard to remember to do tasks outside of our usual routine, so tying a new activity to existing behaviors can help cue us to do it. You might pick right after dinner as the time to reflect and write out your good memory for the day. Or if you have a fitness class three times per week, you might pick the time when you're relaxing after class as good memory-writing time.

4. Write it out. Try to be as specific and detailed as you can. If you heard a new quote that you liked, write out the whole thing on the paper. If you saw a friend in the grocery store, write down their name and a compliment they gave you.

5. Fold your memory up and tuck it in your container.

6. On days when you're feeling low, or any night before bed to put you in a good mood for sleep, pull out one or more memories and revisit them, then put them back into the jar when you're done. You can revisit the same good memory many times!

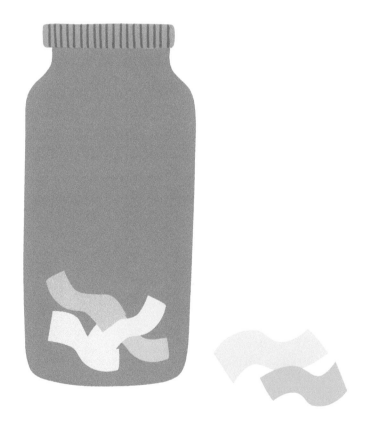

Commercial Breaks That Count

If you're like most of us, you know that commercial breaks during TV shows are a good time to use the restroom or get more snacks. They can also be a prime time to incorporate more stimulating activities into your day and refresh your senses. Believe it or not, watching television can have a number of negative effects on your well-being.

- Sedentary activities like watching television are associated with lower cognitive performance as well as an increased risk of mortality.

- Watching television has been associated with eating more frequently. This is not universal, but it's also not surprising, since many commercials show scrumptious snacks and meals, and their goal is to encourage us to want them.

- TV can reduce melatonin production, a hormone we need to tell our bodies when to go to sleep. A good solution here is to turn off the tube at least an hour before you'd like to fall asleep.

Listed next are several ideas for how to make use of commercial time, so you can skip listening to another pitch about your next snack.

Note: This activity gets a little trickier now that many of our television show–watching methods are commercial-free, but you can still pause the show when the originally planned commercial break would have come on or at your leisure.

NECESSITIES:
A television show on a TV or a laptop

Pick one of these activities to refresh your senses and improve your overall health:

- **Stretch time:** Pick a set of stretches to do during each break, even if it's simply raising your arms above your head, twisting from side to side, and bending down to touch your toes. Repeat.

- **Crunch time:** There's nothing like a short time segment to get in some crunches or leg lifts. See how many you can do during the break, then see if you can beat your record on the next break. (Get physician approval as needed.)

- **Take a breather:** Step outside, breathe in the fresh air, and look at the world around you. It's as simple as that.

- **The 20-20-20 Rule:** Your eyes need a break, too. At least every 20 minutes, focus your eyes on a spot 20 feet away and stare at it for 20 seconds. This allows your eye muscles to relax and refresh.

- **Recap:** See what you recall from the last segment of TV watching. Write down or say aloud the main plot points, any twists and turns, and favorite highlights of the show so far. This will get you in the practice of really thinking about what you're watching.

- **DIY:** Find another activity that offers some cognitive or physical benefit and set your mind to doing it each commercial break. Water your garden, take out your knitting, or make a grocery list for tomorrow.

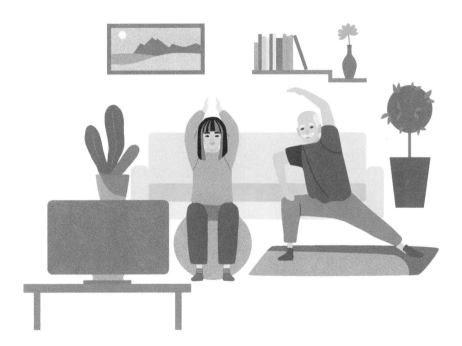

Spark the Conversation

Sometimes we long for human contact, only to find that we're not sure what to say when we finally have company. Here are some discussion prompts that make for great conversation, from small talk to deep reflection. Such social interaction may actually help preserve cognitive function. Depending on how well you know each other or how large the group you're talking to is, you might ask different follow-up questions. These prompts can get people more familiar with each other and sharing new perspectives on life. Write any additional questions you think of in the margins for future conversations.

NECESSITIES:
One or more people, besides you

Pick one or several of the following prompts. These prompts can be taken in a serious or lighthearted way. Get comfy, secure some snacks or a beverage (perhaps some tea from the International Tea Time activity, page 142), and start chatting.

- What's one of your favorite places in the world? What do you like about it?

- When did another person's actions warm your heart?

- If you had to live in cold weather or hot weather for the rest of your life, which would you choose and why?

- What are two things you like about yourself, and when have they helped you or someone else in your life (e.g., sense of humor, work ethic, creativity, etc.)?

- What is one of the activities you have on your bucket list?

- How famous would you like to be before you felt "too famous"?

- What was it like when you moved out of your home for the first time? What helped you find your way?

- What is the first thing you notice about someone you meet?

- If you could eat dinner with two people (famous or ordinary, living or deceased), who would you choose and what would you ask them?

- What was your first pet? What was a favorite pet of yours?

- What character traits do you share with your favorite animal?

- You've just come into $500 million. What would you do?

- If you could send a message to an alien species, what would it be?

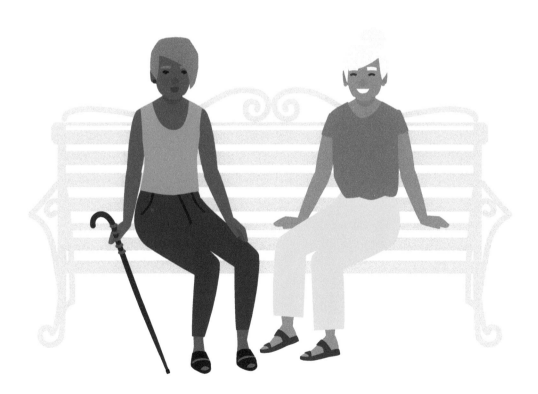

Wanderlust

This activity is designed to stretch your curiosity and planning abilities by organizing a trip to a far-off destination. Even if your traveling has only included nearby spots, you likely know of the planning and organizing required to ensure you have a wonderful time. And if you've traveled extensively, there is bound to be a place on your wish list to explore.

Your task is to do some research based on your interests, pick a location, map out your course, and answer the many questions that come up when planning a trip and traveling. What mode of transportation will you take? Who are your traveling companions? What sights will you see? What activities will you want to try? Be as detailed as you'd like or just take note of the big-picture ideas. The point is to expand your thinking and exercise your organizational skills in a fun way. Perhaps you'll end up planning the perfect trip for the next time you have the urge to get away.

NECESSITIES:

Map (physical or digital, such as Google Maps)

Internet access or a travel book

Pen or pencil (to mark on the map or take notes)

Sticky notes (to post notes on the map)

Scratch paper for notes

1. Select a starting location and find it on your map.

2. Select a destination anywhere in the world and find it on your map.

3. Research the destination online or with a travel book. Don't forget local travel and tourism boards, chambers of commerce, and hyperlocal news and tourism sites and magazines.

4. Consider your interests when you plan your trip. Are you a foodie or a wine connoisseur? Do you like to visit tons of museums and monuments and spend the day walking, or do you like to grab a seat at a coffee shop or a fancy hotel lobby and people watch? This is your trip, so dream big!

5. Once you have the big-picture plans in mind, research the details of your dream trip. Digital tools like TripAdvisor.com or RoadTrippers.com can be helpful. Google Travel has extensive flight and hotel planning capability, and Google Maps and Street View can take you anywhere in the world you want to go, without even leaving your house. Learn what the weather is like at each location you plan to visit. What language is spoken there? What's the food like? What is the history of the destination? What nature or urban experiences do you expect to have? Write these ideas down on sticky notes or scratch paper.

6. Determine if you need a visa to visit your destination and if you would require a translator or guide.

7. Decide how you want to travel—by boat, train, plane, or car, or a mix of these.

8. If you want to expand on your trip, explore possible day trips you might take close to your main destination.

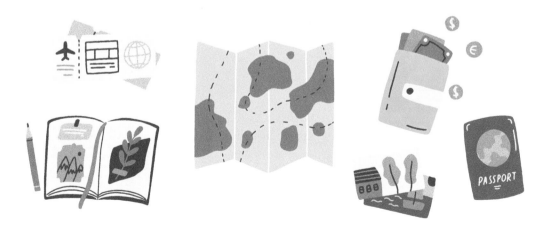

Get Rolling

Rolling clay, that is! Clay is such a forgiving material that you can indulge your creative impulses and not worry too much about do-overs. Feeling relaxed and safe to make mistakes gives our mind the peace it needs to think more clearly. Allow your mind to wander to all of the things you can make out of clay—from coasters and trivets to votive candle holders and chopstick holders. Clay creations can take on any style or message you want, whether sleek, fun, whimsical, feminine, or masculine. It all depends on your choice of textures and shapes.

NECESSITIES:

Clean surface to roll clay out on (a countertop is fine)

Oven-bake clay (any color)

Plastic wrap or nonstick mat

Rolling pin (nonstick or regular, a large can in a pinch)

Cookie cutters, large and small (e.g., circles, stars, squares)

Knife (for cutting off pieces of clay)

Baking pan/dish

Optional: items with surfaces that create added texture, such as a meat tenderizer, leaves, textured fabric, straws, etc. If you're getting really fancy, you can even purchase embossing letters and shapes.

1. Clean and dry your working surface. Lay down a layer of plastic wrap, if you're not using a mat.

2. Place a chunk of clay on your mat/plastic wrap. If using plastic wrap, place another layer on top of the clay so your rolling pin won't stick.

3. Roll out the clay to about ¼-inch thick.

4. Add texture. Place items like leaves or grasses on top of the clay, peeling back the plastic if needed. Roll the rolling pin over them gently to press them into the clay. Remove the objects and observe the texture you created.

5. Using large cookie cutters, stamp your clay. You can stop here and make coasters, or continue and make a votive candle or pen container.

6. If you're making a container, roll out another piece of clay for the sides.

7. Add texture as you did before. For added style, use small stamps or straws to make tiny cutouts in the piece for light to shine through.

8. Cut the pieces to the desired size of your container, keeping the size of the base in mind. For circular containers, cut one piece to wrap around the circular base. For square containers, cut four sides of equal size.

9. Align the edges with the base and each other, then gently brush your fingers across the seams to create a seal.

10. Bake in the oven in an oven-safe baking pan or dish as directed on the clay packaging.

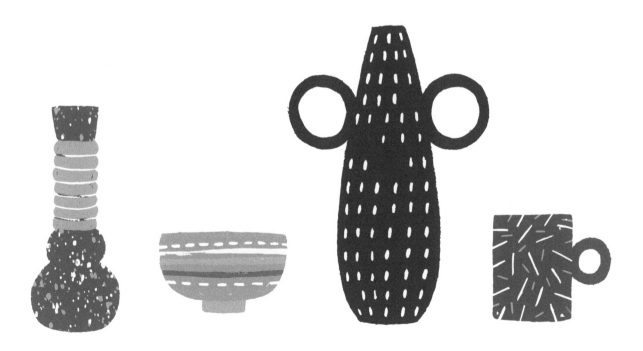

Time Tracing

Life is what happens to you while you're busy making other plans, right? Sometimes the days fly by, while sometimes they seem to repeat.

Even the most monotonous days have some moment that you can highlight, though, and these recollections can help fill in the story of our lives. Traveling through our mental timeline of the last 12 to 24 hours is an excellent way to make sure our recent activities stay fresh in our minds and can help guide our future course of action.

This was actually one of Benjamin Franklin's preferred practices, and he is just one of the many prolific individuals who engaged in a nightly "examination of the day." Revisiting and describing past positive experiences is associated with higher quality of life, plus better cognition and communication. It keeps our minds fresh at orienting to time and pulling up the words to express our thoughts and feelings.

NECESSITIES:

Paper

Pen or pencil

---

1. Decide on your timeframe. Would you rather review the last 8 hours, 24 hours, or week? (Just note that as your timeline gets longer, so can the difficulty in recalling all the little details.)

2. On a blank piece of paper, draw a line from one end of the page to the other. Make marks for each time increment (hours in the day, or days in the week).

3. Look back on the chosen time frame, using any notes you've made and input from loved ones, planners, or calendars. This may be difficult at first, but stick with it. You're exercising your ability to pull details from the past and identify the joys you experience on a regular basis. Referencing your calendar, phone records, or smartphone for location tracking may help jog your memory about where you went and what you did.

4. Now comes the fun and challenging part: Write or draw the places you visited, the people you saw, the scents you smelled, the food you ate, or any other details that stick out to you from this period of time.

5. Circle the items on your list that were your favorite parts—a sight, conversation, person, or experience.

6. Store this page to revisit sometime in the future.

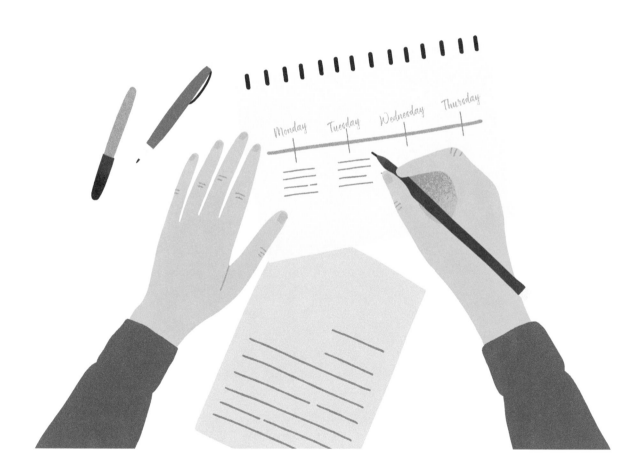

Make Some Scents

One of the most powerful senses that relates to memory is smell. How would we survive without our ability to smell rotten fruit, sour milk, or smoke that warns us of a fire? The smell of a certain perfume, a campfire, or a bouquet of spring flowers can transport us back to a special moment.

One way to harness the experience of scent is to literally wrap it up in individual packages that can be tucked into gym bags, closets, bathroom counters, or car consoles. Depending on the materials you use, these packages can drive away odors while they inspire your senses. You can pick from a range of scents—from floral to woodsy—in this creative activity.

NECESSITIES:

Paper envelopes or sachet bags
  (any size)
Materials for filling (see list below)
Medium bowl

Medium spoon
Ribbon (if sachet bags do not
  already have string/tie on them)
Optional: funnel

FILLING:

10 drops of essential oil (see
  step 2 for options)
2 cups of sachet base (white
  rice or unscented cat litter
  works fine)

Optional: ½ cup lavender buds,
  cedarwood chips, sage leaves,
  or other scented materials

1. Decide how large you'd like each package to be. I choose smaller bags because they fit into more places.

2. Pick up the essential oils and other materials for your filling. Choose your oils based on the mood or effect you'd like them to create. Lavender promotes relaxation, eucalyptus invigorates, rose improves mood and reduces anxiety, rosemary reduces tension and fatigue, and peppermint promotes respiratory and digestive health.

3. In a medium bowl, mix together the base and the essential oil. To make the scent stronger, use more essential oil or less base. Remember not to touch your eyes or your mouth if you get oil on your fingers.

4. Add in any remaining materials you'd like in the sachet, like sage leaves, cedar chips, or dried flowers. Mix well.

5. Using your spoon, scoop the sachet filling into the sachet bags or envelopes. You may wish to use a funnel for this step.

6. Seal the sachet bags by tying the bag's string tightly, or if using envelopes, wetting and closing the seal. Ribbon works well on bags without a string, but make sure to tie it nice and tight so no materials leak out.

7. Place your scented creations wherever you like! Tuck one behind the couch cushion for a pleasant aroma when relaxing, or hand one off to a friend as a gift.

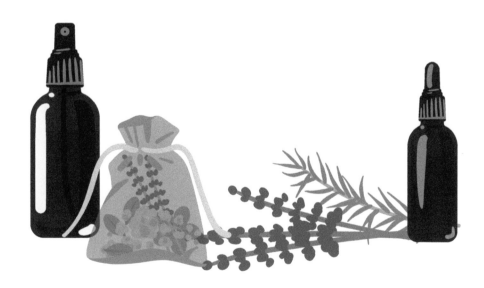

Celebrating Cultures

Whether you're well traveled or not, you can create the flavors and sounds of a day in a different culture. Here in Southern California, we don't have to go far to experience Mexican culture, but I never get tired of creating an immersive experience in my home. Making food and playing music remind me of Mexico's complex history with California and bring me a little closer to parts of my family. Exploring less-familiar cultures can help expand your palate, language skills, knowledge of history, and sense of humanity.

You can opt to explore any culture you'd like, but here, we'll create a dinner experience in the style of Mexican culture. From the vibrant color palette to their spicy dishes, Mexican culture has a typically lively quality with down-to-earth ambiance.

Whether you're already somewhat familiar with or are just being introduced to a new culture, approaching the experience with an open mind can facilitate and deepen your understanding. We can get very used to looking at the world through our own lens, which can be both uncomfortable and refreshing to suspend for a time. The tempo and lyrics of our own music are familiar. That said, you're likely to find shared themes across cultures, such as the emphasis on gathering, sharing a meal, and love lost and found. If possible, gather with family or friends to make this a true cultural celebration!

NECESSITIES:

A few creative touches, perhaps a green, red, and white color scheme to reflect the colors of the Mexican flag

Sound system for playing music

Mexican Music

Mexican food: takeout, or made from scratch

Reading material about Mexican culture

1. Decorate your party space to invoke a feeling of Mexico.

2. Turn on the music. Try the album *Canciones de Mi Padre* by Linda Ronstadt or songs by Julieta Venegas. Also consider mariachi, which is traditional Mexican folk music.

3. Dish up your meal. Try enchiladas, albondigas soup, or tacos. Consider agua fresca for a beverage or a dessert of flan or churros.

4. Read a little about the history of the culture, such as the Aztec legend behind their flag. Take turns reading aloud, if family and friends are joining.

5. Eat, sing, dance, and have a great time!

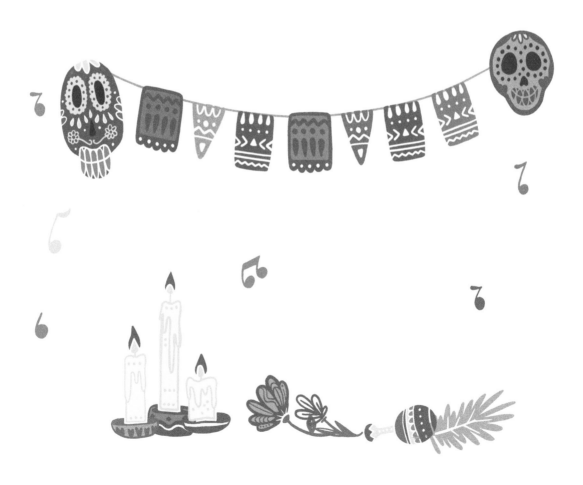

Beanbag Bocce

Bocce (pronounced BAW-chee) is derived from an ancient Roman game and evolved in Italy into a leisurely game of aim and coordination. Bocce starts with throwing out a target ball, then each player on a team throws their ball in turn, trying to land as close to the target ball as possible. It's a great exercise in focus and coordination for the mind and body.

Bocce helps with hand-eye coordination as well as proprioception, or the awareness of the position and movement of your body, as you swivel and direct the ball to the target. As we age, movement can become less automatic and require more conscious effort. As you might guess, engaging in activities that encourage awareness of the position of our joints results in improvement. The "use it or lose it" rule is real here, so why not use it doing a fun outdoor activity?

This game is typically played with firm, roughly baseball-sized balls made of wood, clay, or metal. This makes it somewhat difficult to play on firm or delicate surfaces. Using beanbags that you can easily make at home makes it a more accessible and versatile activity. Fill some old socks with dry rice or beans, and wrap rubber bands around the tops, or sew up the openings. Voilá! You have a set of bocce bags. (You can also find small beanbags at sports equipment stores or online.) Now gather a few friends and head outside for some leisurely competition—or practice solo so you're ready for the next group bocce game!

NECESSITIES:

Beanbags

 4 of one color

 4 of another color

 1 white or black for the target

---

1. Divide into two teams (one to four players per team).

2. The first team throws the target bag, then throws one of their team's bags, trying to land it as close to the target bag as possible.

3. The second team then throws a bag, aiming for the target bag.

4. The teams take turns throwing one bag apiece until all bags are thrown.

5. Once all bags have been thrown, the team whose bag is closest to the target gets a point for that round.

6. If it's a tie, neither team gets a point, or you can flip a coin to see which team gets a point for that round.

7. Continue playing rounds until one team reaches the goal, which is often 13 points. For shorter or longer games, you can adjust the number of goal points accordingly.

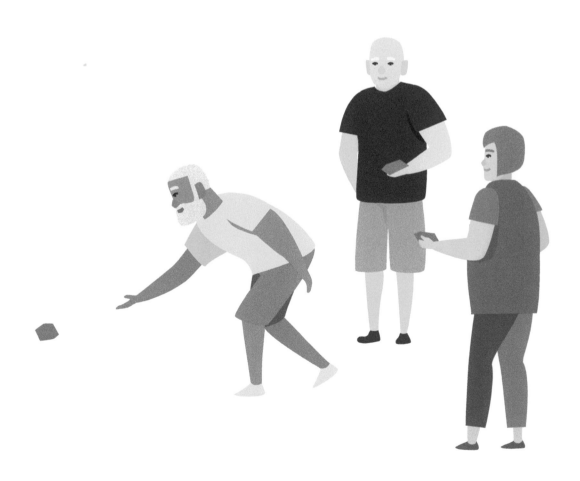

Mascot Photo Tour

Camera-shy folks often have photo libraries filled with landscapes or pictures of food without a consistent subject—in this case a person—linking them together. Scenery can indeed be beautiful, but adding someone or something that ties snapshots together in a fun, creative way is a great method to exercise your mind.

This activity is inspired by the movie *Amélie*, where the main character, Amélie, creates a series of photos using a garden gnome as the "traveler." Now it's your turn to pick your own traveler, or mascot. It can be a bobblehead, figurine, mug with a face on it, or even your pet. Now plan some adventures out on the town or in nature, and arrange to capture your subject on camera. This is a great excuse to visit new sites, create fun and interesting scenes to photograph, and tell a new story with your mascot as the main character. If anyone questions what you are up to, you can honestly tell them with a smile: "I'm creating art."

NECESSITIES:
Camera

Mascot

1. Locate your camera.

2. Decide on a mascot for a subject.

3. Find various places to stage your mascot and start snapping pictures. You can begin in your home, then venture out to parks, cafés, or neighborhood venues if you'd like. If someone normally accompanies you out of the house, make sure they're on board with your plans and can go along to help with setup.

4. Let your mascot explore the heights and depths of their new world. Just be sure they—and you!—don't fall from a ledge or into a hole where they can't easily be recovered. Consider tying a string to your

mascot that you can hold while they are placed in any precarious poses. And of course, if your live pet is your mascot, stick to the safer positions.

5. See what emotions you can evoke with your settings and poses. Maybe you have your mascot playing in a pile of fall leaves, or peeking out from behind a tree in the distance to suggest secrecy or shyness.

6. Depending on your camera setup—a phone camera, a point-and-shoot, or a DSLR—play with color and filters. Make a statement by turning the photo black and white, or add a nostalgic feel with a sepia filter. Photo-editing computer programs and smartphone apps offer endless opportunities to improve and adjust your images, or even add text and borders if you're feeling extra creative.

7. Consider printing the photos and using them to illustrate your stories from two other activities in this book: Write Your Story (page 198) or Family Storyboard (page 196). You're taking a number of pictures that share the theme of your selected mascot, making them a fine foundation for a photo story. Pin your prints to a board for a short photo sequence, make a collage, or just flip through them every so often and have a laugh.

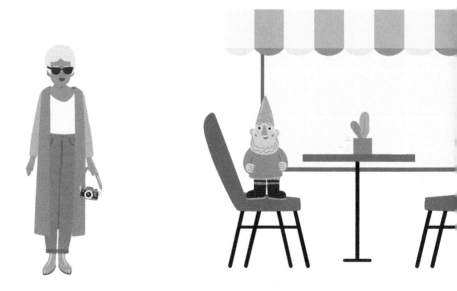

A Tourist in Your Town

I spent months living in the same city, only to one day pick up a tourist map and find I hadn't visited more than 20 percent of the suggested attractions. A friend and I decided it was time to acquaint ourselves with our local must-see places and activities, and it turned out to be one of my most memorable days there. Strolling to the next location on the map made me feel like a tourist in my own town, and took me to places I likely would never have sought out on my own.

Discovery of and exposure to new locations fuel creativity and brain activity, as our brains work to accommodate new sights, smells, and sounds. Stop by your local chamber of commerce or city center for a guide to your city, download one online and print it, or use a travel guide app on your phone. Get ready for a day of discovery and feel like a tourist close to home. Remember to take plenty of photos of your experience, especially when you discover a new favorite spot. Have fun exploring!

NECESSITIES:

Printed local map or smartphone map app

Optional: Snacks (see step 3)

---

1. Locate a map of local sites. Use guides and/or walking tours with a variety of interesting local landmarks, historic locations, cultural or natural attractions, neighborhoods, activities, and restaurants.

2. Schedule out the day. Gauge the distances between the sites you want to visit. Do you only want to be out for a few hours, or all day? Consider splitting up your trips to the sites you want to visit over a few days or weeks.

3. Bring snacks, such as an apple, some almonds, or other energy-smart foods that will tide you over until your next meal, so you will have enough energy to focus on your adventure. Alternatively, pick a great restaurant in town that offers a unique culinary experience to add to your agenda.

4. Pick up mementos as you explore. If you're the type to scrapbook or keep some memorabilia on your dresser from a neat new locale, bring home that funny-looking leaf or support your local economy and buy that cool sticker. Just be sure to respect the local habitat.

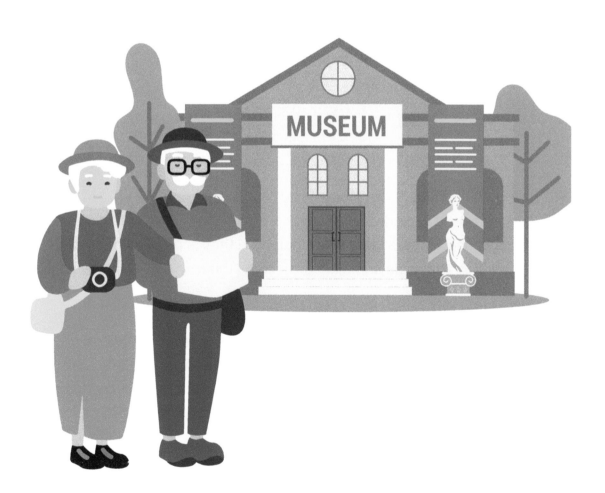

The Memory Card Game

Give your spatial memory a workout while having some friendly competition! This classic game—built around which player can collect the most pairs of matching cards—engages your short- and long-term memory. It relies on you tracking where the matching cards lie among a grid of face-down cards. This can be a bit tricky but can be adapted to be easier to play.

Have you ever reorganized your toolbox or spice rack only to be a little confused for a while until you oriented to the new location of everything? This straightforward yet at times tricky game is like a shot of that, exercising your ability in retaining the location of each card while hunting for its counterpart. And if you play multiple games in a row, you have to refresh your mental map in order to have the latest location of the card—an engaging and stimulating task!

NECESSITIES:

Deck of cards

Flat playing space, such as a table or the floor

1. Lay out a deck of cards in rows and columns (forming a square). For easier or shorter play, remove two pairs at a time (e.g., two Jacks) from the deck so you're playing with fewer cards total.

2. Take turns with one or more people flipping over two cards at a time.

3. If both cards flipped on one turn match (same value and color), put them in your winning pile to be counted at the end of the game. Leave the rest of the cards where they lie and continue playing. If they don't match, turn them both back over, and it's the next player's turn.

4. Be sure to pay attention to which cards your opponent flips over on their turn as well as your own. All flips are insight into where the various cards lie.

5. Once no cards are left on the table, you each count up your cards.

6. Whoever has the most cards wins!

7. Feel free to play this game solo as a means of exercising your memory. You can even see how few turns you can take to gather all the cards and set a personal record. You can also practice motor speed by setting a timer to see if you can beat your previous time.

8. Whether you play alone or with a partner, see what strategies help you recall the location of each card. Perhaps you can visualize the grid right to left or make patterns out of the locations of the cards, like constellations. Use your imagination!

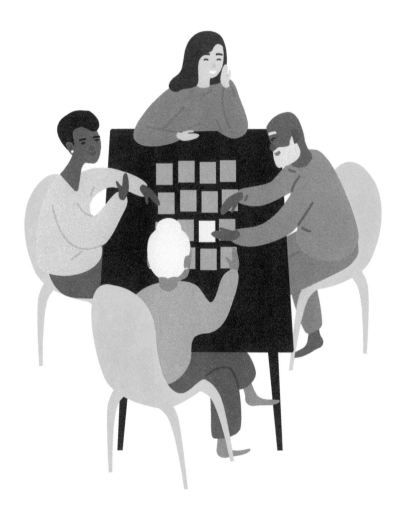

Green Thumbs Up

Bring some nature into your life by creating a succulent garden wreath. This activity challenges your visual-spatial and fine motor skills, while you craft a dramatic and earthy presentation that will live for months.

Whether or not you have a green thumb, low-maintenance succulents will work for anyone. You can arrange them partially around a wreath or in a full circle. Most of the materials are typically found at craft stores or nurseries. Succulents come in so many sizes, shapes, and hues that choosing the perfect plants for your design will be a fun and creative exercise, too. Allow your creativity to flow as you nestle each succulent cutting within the larger arrangement.

NECESSITIES:

Succulent cuttings (small and large flower-sized pieces)

Wreath branches (such as willow or grapevine) or a premade grapevine wreath

Moss (sphagnum/peat moss)

Raffia or brown twine

Tacky glue

Optional: spray bottle for watering

If you're having trouble envisioning these steps, try searching for "succulent wreath" videos online. There are good demonstrations on various ways to construct your own version of this wreath.

1. Make the succulent cuttings one to two days ahead of time so they have a chance to dry over the cut portions.

2. Weave the branches into a circle to make the wreath. Tuck in the loose ends and tie with twine every six inches or so to hold the branches in place.

3. Place mounds of peat moss on the wreath where you'd like the succulents to be located.

4. Tie a long piece of twine around the branches to anchor the moss to the wreath. Then wrap the twine around the moss and branches like a candy cane stripe, leaving 1- to 2-inch gaps, to hold the moss in place. Wrap back in the opposite direction for added support.

5. Using your finger or a pencil, push a small hole in the moss where you'd like to place your succulent. Place each succulent over the holes to test out your arrangement.

6. Once you have an arrangement you like, fill each hole with tacky glue, then place the succulent back in the hole. Let the wreath rest for at least one hour to let the glue dry.

7. Place or hang the wreath in a slightly shady place.

8. Every week or two, water your succulents by heavily spritzing the moss. Mark on the calendar which day(s) of the week/month it needs to be watered.

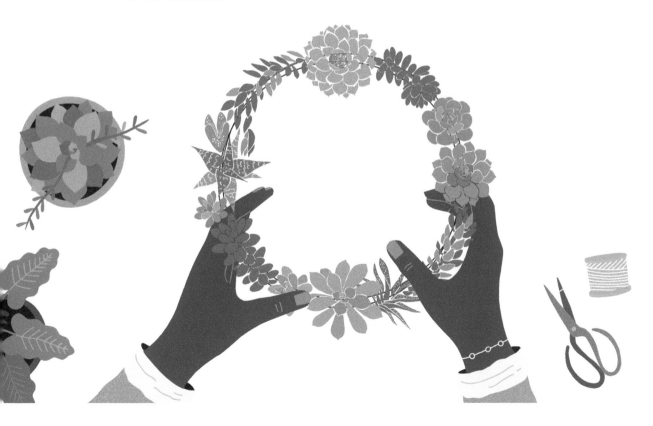

Cookies Around the World

Cookies are believed to originate from the increasing use of sugar in seventh-century Persia. They were later brought to Europe, eventually becoming a delicious treat in countries around the globe. Like bread, cookies appear in various forms in many cultures, with each putting their spin on this sweet treat. Textures range from buttery melt-in-your-mouth crumbles found in the Russian tea cake to the chewy crispness of Australia's Anzac biscuits.

Challenge your cognitive skills and explore world cultures by seeking out recipes for cookies from different places, baking a batch (or six), and sharing with a friend. If baking isn't your thing, you can pick them up at a brick-and-mortar or online grocery store, specialty food market, or ethnic restaurant or bakery. The important thing is to enjoy this sweet culinary history lesson and invite a friend to join you.

NECESSITIES:

Cookies

Optional: recipe for one of the cookies covered on the next page

---

1. Pick up at the market one or more of the three cookies from around the world listed on the next page, or make them at home for a more active, mentally engaging experience. Recipes (such as those found at food blogs like Cooking.NYTimes.com or AheadOfThyme.com) provide the steps for challenging your mind to organize the timing, ratios, and mechanics of baking.

2. Read up on the history and symbolism of the cookies within their culture.

3. Enjoy these cookies with a friend while sharing the wonderful heritage of these sweet treats, perhaps pairing them with some tea from the International Tea Time activity on page 142.

- **Persian Nan-e Nokhodchi (noon-eh-khohd-chee):** Given the origin of cookies, it only seems natural to start with this delicate and delicious chickpea flour cookie from Persian culture. These bite-sized morsels are commonly made during Nowruz (the Persian New Year celebrations) and placed on the sofreh (meaning "table") in the Haft-seen, which is a display of seven symbols of nature and renewal.

- **Dutch Speculaas (speck-ooh-lass):** The Dutch blessed (what would become) the United States with koekjes in New Amsterdam in the late 1620s, where "koekje" was eventually Anglicized to "cookie." Speculaas (or, for Belgian-Dutch, "speculoos") are flat, thin, and crisp and traditionally come in the shape of a windmill, but more commonly are rectangular-shaped. These spiced delights are made for the Feast of St. Nicholas in the Netherlands, Belgium, Germany, and Austria.

- **Italian Biscotti (bee-SKAW-tee):** Their name is the Italian word for "twice cooked." Originally carried by Roman legions into battle and hailing more specifically from Tuscany (a region in Italy), these long, crisp cookies make excellent material for dunking (think coffee or tea). Nowadays, these crunchy cookies come in a variety of flavors and are often partially dipped in chocolate.

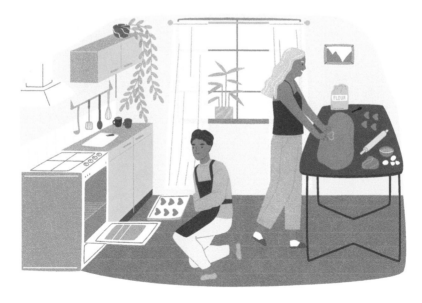

Your Other Half

Games can entertain us and sharpen our wits and mental faculties at the same time. This active and approachable game for all ages works well as a stimulating activity for medium to large parties. It's a quick game of acting, listening, and locating, with pairs racing to identify their partner who shares the same cue. It can be made more complex by having pairs impersonate famous people. Get ready to keep your eyes and ears peeled in this lively and social game!

NECESSITIES:

Group of 8 or more people

Pen or pencil

Small pieces of paper

Bowl or hat

1. Write items to be sung, spoken, or sounded out on the pieces of paper. This might be a list of well-known songs, famous quotes, or animals (for their sounds). Write two of each item (e.g., two pieces of paper that have "*Rocky* Theme" written on them).

2. Write as many item pairs as needed so that each person can get one piece of paper. For instance, if there are 8 people, you'll only need 4 item pairs. If you have an odd number of people, the odd person out can take turns leading the players.

3. Put the pieces of paper in a bowl or a hat and mix thoroughly.

4. Each person picks a piece of paper, reads it, and keeps their cue a secret. They can hold on to their paper for the rest of that round.

5. The leader designates a "home base" (usually a wall to touch or a threshold/doorway to cross).

6. Everyone then gathers in the middle of the room. When the leader says "go," everyone begins saying or singing their item.

7. Each person listens for their partner—someone singing or saying the same thing as they are. When they find them, they grab hands and touch "home base" (the designated wall). If speed and/or mobility is an issue, you can alternatively have pairs grab hands and hold them up together as a symbol of their success in finding each other.

8. The last pair to reach "home base" together is out for the remaining rounds of that game. The rounds continue until there is one winning pair left standing.

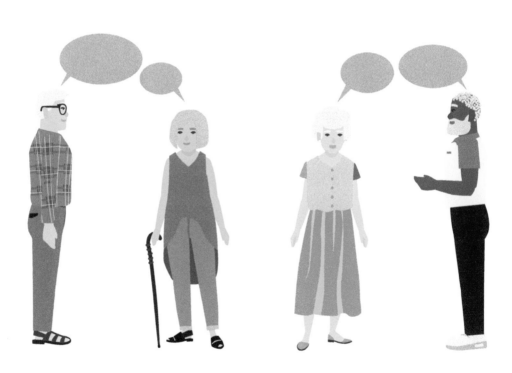

News Clues

Often there's a great news story I'm inspired to share with a friend, only to wonder silently to myself how the details lined up. If you've ever had a similar experience, then this activity is for you. Give your memory a leg up by putting together a news synopsis gallery of all your favorite news stories. Follow the stories over time, noting which details emerge and when. Later, review this treasure trove of facts about anything from nature to human interest stories.

This activity flexes many mental muscles, including memory, selective attention, and organization, while you compile and reflect on your selected stories.

Note: The news can be a place of wonder and inspiration, as well as tragedy and suffering. Striking a balance by being selective of which stories you choose to follow can help direct the impact of news on your mood.

NECESSITIES:

News access (e.g., newspaper or online newsfeed)

Notebook and binder or a computer document (e.g., spreadsheet or document)

---

1. Spend a few minutes on a regular basis, such as daily or Sunday mornings, reading through your news source.

2. Save each story that holds your interest by first writing down the topic in your notebook or computer document.

3. Next, summarize the main points of the article. What are the takeaways you hope to recall or might say during a short conversation with a friend? Who are the main characters involved?

4. Save photos to your document or cut them out from the paper to put in your binder.

5. You can sort stories into sections (e.g., nature, finance, etc.) using a binder or digital tabs.

6. As you continue to read the news over weeks and months, add developments to your notebook by placing the date where you left off for that topic and jotting down the new details.

7. Review your news clues whenever you want a refresher, or quiz yourself by reading just the topic and attempting to recall as many details from memory as you can.

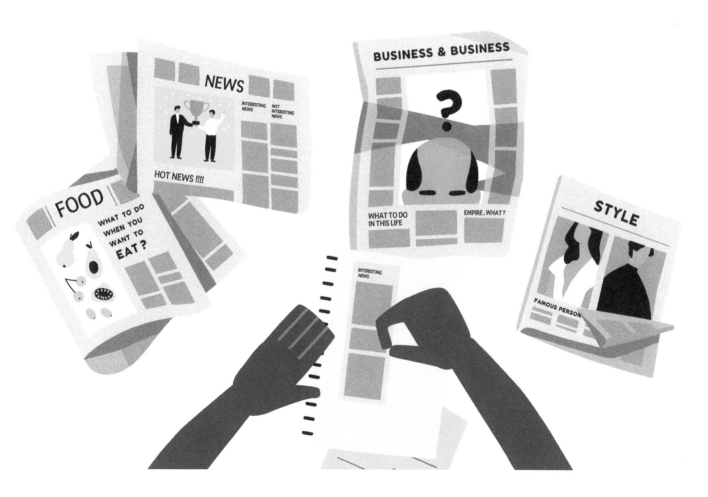

Write a Song

Music has some magical effects on brain health. These have been studied in depth, notably by the neurologist Oliver Sacks in his book *Musicophilia*.

Do you ever notice how you can't recall all the lyrics to a song, but after being given just a few beats and the first words, the rest comes rushing to your mind? Dr. Sacks discovered in working with individuals with amnesia following brain injury that music can call moments and abilities to our minds that we thought were lost forever.

Music affects the everyday thinker quite similarly. It's a dynamic force that elicits rhythmic sensation, social engagement, and emotional charge. Believe it or not, these are all things that assist memory! Turn on the song you heard in your first year of junior high school, and your experience of that long-ago moment will likely come to mind more clearly. Song lyrics often have a chorus, which repeats and facilitates memory. That's why you'll see most people singing along to the chorus. Song verses are sections of words that change from the beginning to the end of the song, making them a bit harder to remember.

You may have written a song before, or maybe this is a new activity for you. You can keep the first attempt simple and rewrite the lyrics to an old tune, for example, the tune of "Yellow Submarine" by the Beatles, or of a favorite song.

NECESSITIES:

Paper

Pen or pencil

Optional: rhythm instrument/shaker, tambourine, etc.

1. Pick a topic. You can write about the past (a good way to remember past events), the present (e.g., your current feelings), or the future (e.g., something you're anticipating). Or write about a concept or activity, such as love or cooking.

2. Jot down some lyrics. Lyrics don't have to be complex to be enjoyable. Throw down a few lines that express just how you think or feel about something.

3. Rhyme it if you'd like—or not! (e.g., "Ooh, baby, do you know what that's worth? Ooh, heaven is a place on earth.")

4. Use non-word sounds (e.g., "Nah nah nah nah, hey, hey, good bye.")

5. Play your song. Sing it out loud to a beat, or hum it to yourself while saying the lyrics in your mind.

6. If you or a friend play an instrument and you'd like to take it to the next level, compose the instrumental music for your song, using background chords, a clear melody, or both.

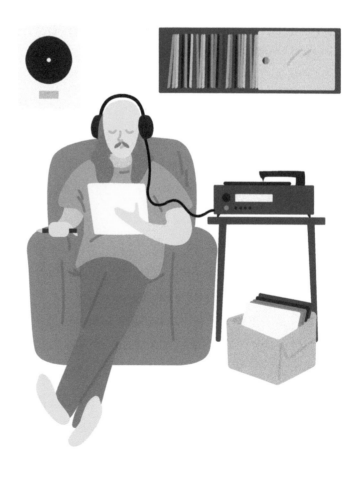

Family Storyboard

Storyboards are like little comic strips featuring approximately six to ten frames that link together to tell a story. This is a creative way to present family stories and can be as simple or complex as you'd like, challenging your memory, organization, and more. Share an amazing day at the beach your family had last summer or a more sentimental memory, such as how you and your partner met. Each frame shares a scene of this experience from start to finish.

Creating a storyboard is easy, and you don't have to be talented at drawing to make one. You can keep it simple by drawing stick figures or gluing down photographs. Each person involved will likely remember their own version of the same experience. Piece together your story from your family's or friends' memories, or create a storyboard based exclusively on your personal memories of an experience.

Gather print or digital family photographs, and determine which scenes are important for capturing the steps of the story. Then put it down in a storyboard format, and reminisce about sentimental moments and fun times. Who knows, maybe this will be your next holiday greeting card!

NECESSITIES:

Large card stock or heavy paper (11" x 17" is a nice size)
Pen or pencil

Optional: photos, glue stick, colored markers

1. Decide on a story. Try to pick one that has a few memorable twists and turns. For example, the time the car broke down during that trip to the mountains. Refer to some comics for inspiration on how to present your family's story. You can find them in the Sunday paper or in an online search.

2. Write out the main scenes of your story that come to mind. For instance, scene one: packing the car; scene two: everyone listening to Mom's cheesy love songs and feigning annoyance but actually liking

them; and scene three: the car breaks down. Sketch out all of your frames, up to ten if you'd like.

3. Now create the graphics for each scene/frame. You can stick to stick figures, glue some printed photos to the board, or go for full illustrations if you'd like.

4. Make use of sound effects and speech bubbles for a more descriptive, lively story. Incorporate any thought bubbles, speech bubbles, or sound effects into the scenes, like a "Pow!" sound effect coming out from the hood of the car. You can draw these, add them in a presentation software such as PowerPoint or Pages, purchase them as stickers from a craft supply store, or add to a digital photo with an app such as PicMonkey or Canva.

5. If you feel like a frame needs a little more explanation, write a sentence or two underneath to elaborate on the meaning of the scene for the viewer.

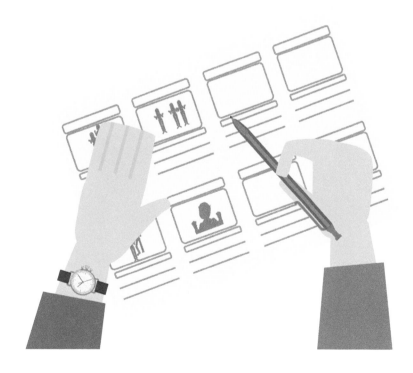

Write Your Story

You're not a writer, you say? Thankfully this isn't a competition—it's simply a way to flex that creativity "muscle" in your brain. In doing so, you also train your brain to organize information.

You can draw from a real-life experience or make up a fictional character and plot. Consider using the Write a Song activity (page 194) or the Mascot Photo Tour activity (page 180) as material for your story. You can write a five-sentence short story or a saga that you return to for "the next episode" with the same main characters. Get your ideas onto the page without being too critical of the exact details or structure. If you enjoy telling the story, and there's a beginning, middle, and end, you're doing just great!

NECESSITIES:

Pen and paper or computer

---

1. Gather your writing materials. Begin by writing down a few ideas on what might be fun or interesting to write about. List real-life experiences or fictional plots.

2. Alternatively, use one of the following plots:

   - A city-dweller inherits a horse ranch.

   - Two people are stranded after a plane wreck.

   - A dog finds out he's going to a new owner.

   - A person starts their own food truck, but runs into some hiccups.

   - A family travels by train to the other side of the country.

   As you can see, each plot has a point of tension requiring some resolution. Will everything work out in the end? That's for you to write out. Any good story has an unknown ending with a plot that unfolds and fills in as the story progresses.

3. Pick the main character(s) and give them some personality through their thoughts, decisions, and reactions. What do they look like? What are their hopes? What are their strengths and weaknesses?

4. Describe the obstacles your characters face. Fill in the little details. What's difficult for them? Does anyone or anything help them along the way?

5. How does the story end? Is it a cliffhanger? Do the characters grow in some way from their experiences? Remember, there's no right way to end it.

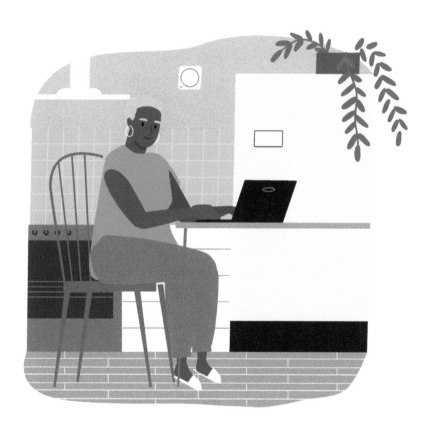

Roll 'Em!

There are a number of dice games out there, but this one in particular comes to mind because it requires some thinking power. Originally appearing as Pocket Farkel in the mid-1980s, it's also known as Dice 10,000, Hot Dice, and Squelch, among other names. It can be played with two or more players and takes about 20 minutes. Each player takes a turn rolling the dice to collect more points (see point key graphic on the next page).

As the game progresses, you risk losing points from your existing roll to chance gaining more. You'll use your cognitive skills by tracking how many points you have waiting for you to put in the bank, or to risk losing that turn if you toss a losing roll.

NECESSITIES:

One or more other people
6 standard dice
Paper

Pen or Pencil
Dice key (see next page)

---

1. Pick who rolls all six dice first (whose birthday falls earliest in the month or whoever rolls the highest single die).

2. Count up the points using the dice key, then choose to either "bank" those points and hand the dice to the next player or continue rolling and risk losing all points earned so far for that turn.

3. Bank your points by writing the total for that roll under your name on a piece of paper, or really challenge your memory and play by the honor system using mental math! Any dice left that don't contribute to your banked points can be rolled by the next player who starts with the points you banked.

4. If you keep rolling, you pick up and re-roll any dice that aren't creating points, such as a lone 3 or 4.

5. If all dice are contributing points, then you can pick all the dice up again and roll for even more points. Be sure to keep a running tally in your head or on paper.

6. If you roll and none of the dice rolled earn you additional points, your turn is over, you lose all points for that round, and the dice get passed to the next player.

7. The player who reaches 10,000 points first wins!

8. It may take a minute to get the hang of this one, but once you do it's a fun and portable pastime.

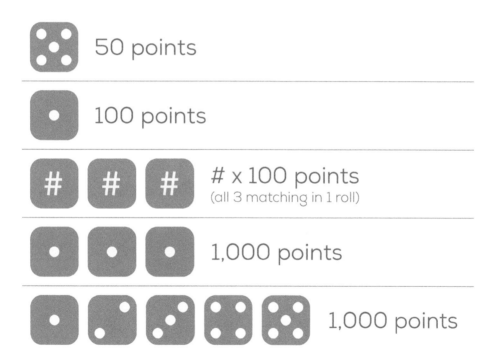

50 points

100 points

x 100 points
(all 3 matching in 1 roll)

1,000 points

1,000 points

ANSWERS: CHAPTER 2

CHALLENGE LEVEL 1

Crosswords

DAYS OF THE WEEK

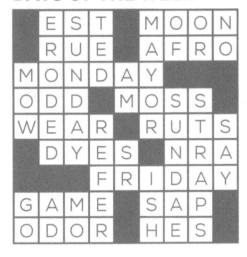

POPULAR SPORTS

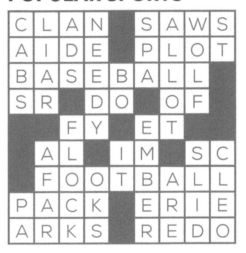

BIG ANIMALS

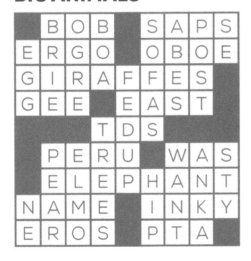

PUBLIC PLACES

WEATHER FORECASTS

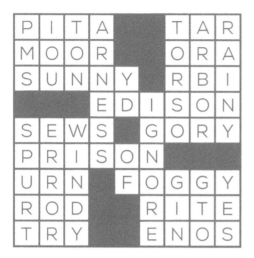

PEOPLE WITH PROFESSIONS

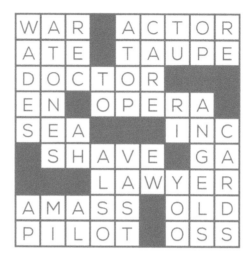

Word Searches

THE ANIMAL KINGDOM

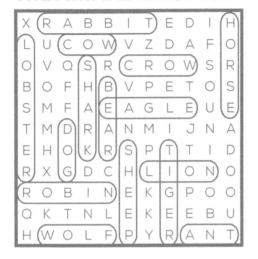

FOOTWEAR

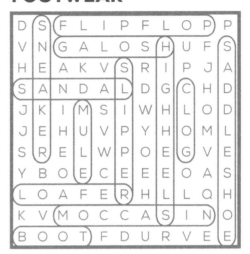

ROUND THINGS

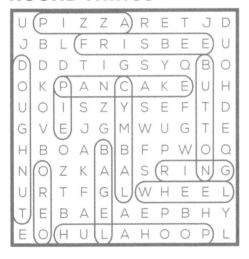

AT THE BEACH

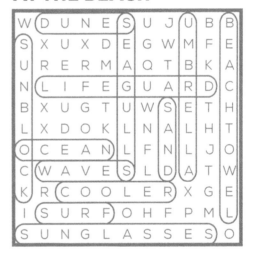

GAMBLING GAMES

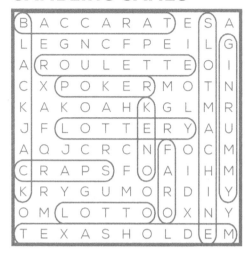

PARTS OF THE BODY

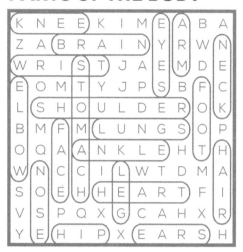

Word Scrambles

WHAT'S FOR DINNER?

1. steak
2. potatoes
3. peas
4. carrots
5. bread
6. butter
7. salad
8. apple pie

DO I HEAR MUSIC?

1. piano
2. violin
3. harp
4. guitar
5. drums
6. flute
7. trumpet
8. trombone

NAME THAT PRESIDENT

1. Lincoln
2. Taft
3. Wilson
4. Truman
5. Kennedy
6. Nixon
7. Ford
8. Obama

Double Word Scrambles

COLORS

1. pink
2. white
3. brown
4. orange
   Bonus: RAINBOW

BIRDS

1. duck
2. eagle
3. goose
4. pigeon
   Bonus: GOLDEN EGG

CLOTHES

1. dress
2. pants
3. shirt
4. jacket
   Bonus: SERAPE

CHALLENGE LEVEL 2

Crosswords

ON THE MONEY

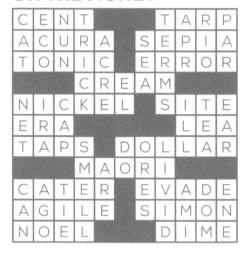

HEALTHY THINGS TO DO

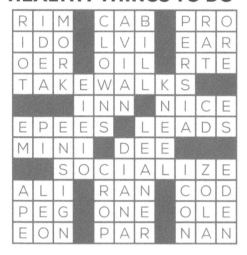

WHAT'S STORED IN THE GARAGE?

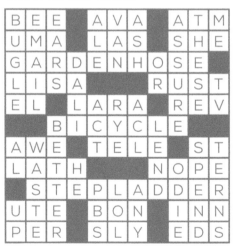

A MORNING RITUAL

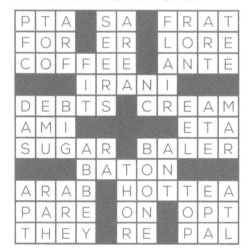

CARD GAMES

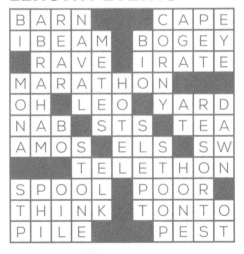

PAPER THINGS

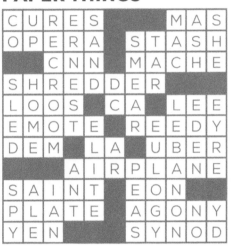

LENGTHY EVENTS

Word Searches

POPULAR SPORTS

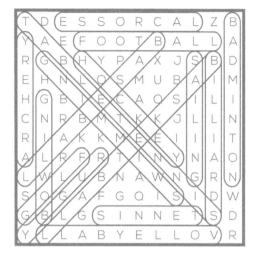

20TH-CENTURY ARTISTS

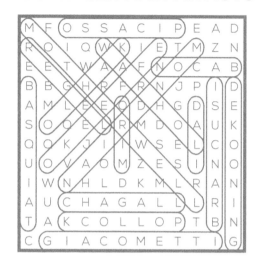

ON THE DANCE FLOOR

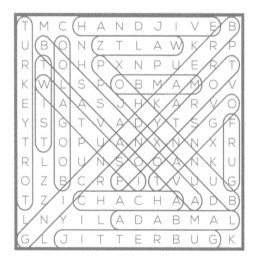

MODERN INVENTIONS

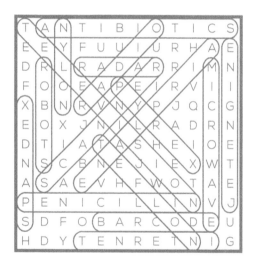

WHAT'S THE WEATHER LIKE TODAY?

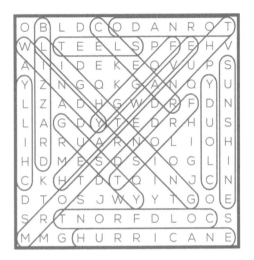

FOOTBALL ACTION

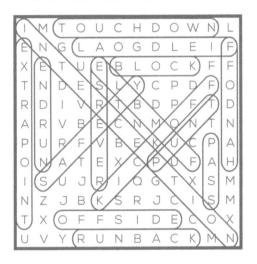

Word Scrambles

GEMSTONES

1. diamond
2. ruby
3. pearl
4. emerald
5. topaz
6. opal
7. spinel
8. sapphire
9. amethyst

A HANDYMAN'S TOOLS

1. hammer
2. nails
3. pliers
4. clamp
5. drill
6. level
7. screws
8. wrench
9. duct tape

THIS OLD HOUSE

1. windows
2. doors
3. roof
4. attic
5. garage
6. stairs
7. porch
8. chimney
9. basement

Double Word Scrambles

OFFICE SUPPLIES

1. paste
2. stamps
3. eraser
4. pencil
   Bonus: PAPER CLIP

FLOWERS

1. pansy
2. peony
3. crocus
4. violet
   Bonus: (a) ROSE (b) TULIP

MAKES OF CARS

1. Acura
2. Buick
3. Honda
4. Toyota
   Bonus: AUTOBAHN

CHALLENGE LEVEL 3

Crosswords

BASEBALL

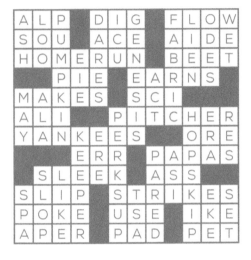

A	L	P		D	I	G			F	L	O	W
S	O	U		A	C	E		A	I	D	E	
H	O	M	E	R	U	N		B	E	E	T	
		P	I	E		E	A	R	N	S		
M	A	K	E	S		S	C	I				
A	L	I			P	I	T	C	H	E	R	
Y	A	N	K	E	E	S		O	R	E		
		E	R	R		P	A	P	A	S		
	S	L	E	E	K		A	S	S			
S	L	I	P		S	T	R	I	K	E	S	
P	O	K	E		U	S	E		I	K	E	
A	P	E	R		P	A	D		P	E	T	

THE SILVER SCREEN

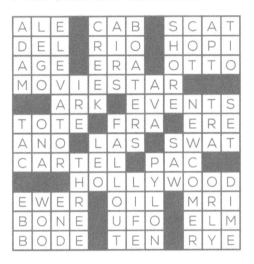

A	L	E		C	A	B		S	C	A	T	
D	E	L		R	I	O		H	O	P	I	
A	G	E		E	R	A		O	T	T	O	
M	O	V	I	E	S	T	A	R				
		A	R	K		E	V	E	N	T	S	
T	O	T	E		F	R	A		E	R	E	
A	N	O		L	A	S		S	W	A	T	
C	A	R	T	E	L		P	A	C			
		H	O	L	L	Y	W	O	O	D		
E	W	E	R		O	I	L		M	R	I	
B	O	N	E		U	F	O		E	L	M	
B	O	D	E		T	E	N		R	Y	E	

MOTTO

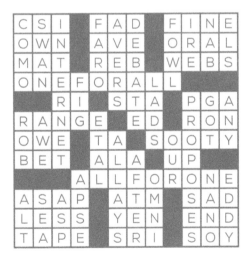

C	S	I		F	A	D		F	I	N	E	
O	W	N		A	V	E		O	R	A	L	
M	A	T		R	E	B		W	E	B	S	
O	N	E	F	O	R	A	L	L				
		R	I		S	T	A		P	G	A	
R	A	N	G	E		E	D		R	O	N	
O	W	E		T	A		S	O	O	T	Y	
B	E	T		A	L	A		U	P			
		A	L	L	F	O	R	O	N	E		
A	S	A	P		A	T	M		S	A	D	
L	E	S	S		Y	E	N		E	N	D	
T	A	P	E		S	R	I		S	O	Y	

BACK IN THE DAY

P	O	W		P	A	S		T	S	P		
S	K	I	D		A	S	P		T	A	K	E
S	A	M	E		P	T	A		U	N	I	T
T	Y	P	E	W	R	I	T	E	R			
		R	O	I		E	M	B	A	L	M	
	C	H	E	E	K	S		S	O	F	I	A
B	O	O		A	B	E		A	N	Y		
A	L	U	M	S		A	M	P	E	R	E	
A	E	R	A	T	E		P	I	T			
	F	A	X	M	A	C	H	I	N	E		
S	A	R	I		E	O	N		E	D	I	E
A	R	E	A		R	U	E		R	O	L	L
G	E	T			T	E	L			L	E	S

212   Answers: Chapter 2

A WALK DOWN
MEMORY LANE

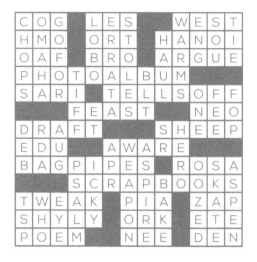

SUNNY SIDE UP

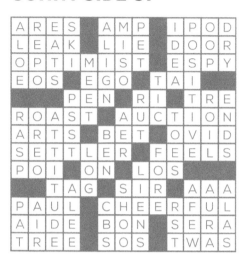

Word Searches

CAR PARTS

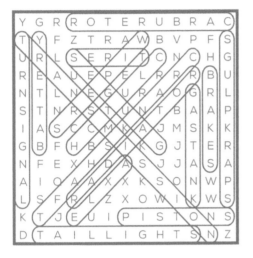

POCKET FULL OF POSIES

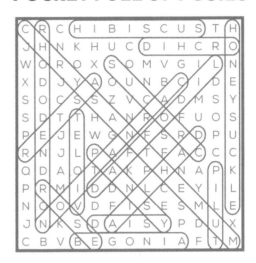

COLORFUL COLORS

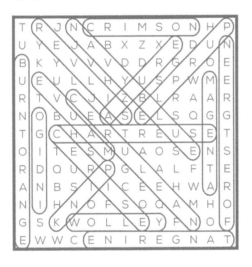

2019 NCAA "SWEET SIXTEEN" TEAMS

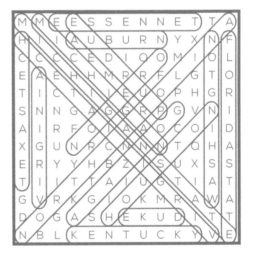

SYNONYMS FOR "CAREFUL"

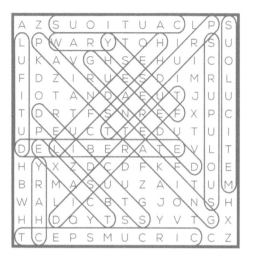

THE 15 LARGEST STATES, AND THE SMALLEST STATE (BY AREA)

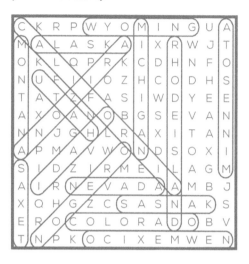

Word Scrambles

GREEN VEGGIES

1. celery
2. endive
3. kale
4. cabbage
5. lettuce
6. parsley
7. arugula
8. cucumber
9. broccoli
10. zucchini

EASTERN U.S. STATES

1. Vermont
2. Maine
3. Ohio
4. Florida
5. Alabama
6. Georgia
7. Indiana
8. Maryland
9. Kentucky
10. Michigan

TOP U.S. COLLEGES

1. Harvard
2. Emory
3. Yale
4. Brown
5. Cornell
6. Rutgers
7. Princeton
8. Columbia
9. Stanford
10. Dartmouth

Double Word Scrambles

TREES

1. cedar
2. willow
3. spruce
4. dogwood
   Bonus: REDWOOD

BIRDS

1. stork
2. finch
3. swallow
4. seagull
   Bonus: OSTRICH

UNITED NATIONS MEMBER COUNTRIES

1. Sweden
2. Kuwait
3. Estonia
4. Hungary
   Bonus: SOUTH SUDAN

ANSWERS: CHAPTER 3

Sudokus

SUDOKU 1

9	7	5	1	6	3	8	2	4
1	6	8	4	9	2	7	3	5
4	3	2	5	8	7	6	9	1
2	9	1	3	7	6	5	4	8
8	4	7	2	1	5	9	6	3
6	5	3	8	4	9	2	1	7
7	2	4	9	5	1	3	8	6
3	8	6	7	2	4	1	5	9
5	1	9	6	3	8	4	7	2

SUDOKU 3

2	7	6	5	1	4	9	8	3
4	3	5	2	8	9	6	7	1
1	8	9	6	3	7	5	4	2
3	6	4	9	7	1	2	5	8
8	5	1	3	2	6	7	9	4
7	9	2	8	4	5	3	1	6
9	4	8	7	6	3	1	2	5
6	1	7	4	5	2	8	3	9
5	2	3	1	9	8	4	6	7

SUDOKU 2

1	5	3	9	6	2	7	4	8
9	4	7	8	1	5	2	6	3
6	2	8	3	7	4	1	9	5
2	6	1	5	4	8	9	3	7
8	7	9	1	2	3	6	5	4
5	3	4	6	9	7	8	1	2
3	9	5	2	8	6	4	7	1
7	1	2	4	3	9	5	8	6
4	8	6	7	5	1	3	2	9

SUDOKU 4

6	4	9	3	8	2	1	5	7
5	8	3	9	7	1	6	2	4
7	2	1	6	4	5	9	3	8
2	3	5	1	6	7	8	4	9
1	6	8	5	9	4	3	7	2
9	7	4	8	2	3	5	1	6
8	1	7	2	5	6	4	9	3
3	9	2	4	1	8	7	6	5
4	5	6	7	3	9	2	8	1

SUDOKU 5

4	5	6	8	9	7	1	3	2
1	2	9	4	3	6	8	5	7
3	7	8	5	2	1	9	6	4
8	4	2	7	6	9	5	1	3
7	9	3	2	1	5	4	8	6
5	6	1	3	8	4	2	7	9
9	8	5	6	7	2	3	4	1
2	3	7	1	4	8	6	9	5
6	1	4	9	5	3	7	2	8

Number Searches

NUMBER SEARCH 1

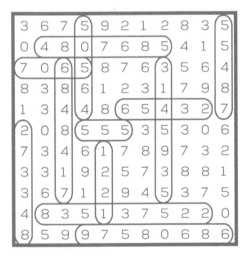

NUMBER SEARCH 2

NUMBER SEARCH 3

```
9  5  5  6  7  2  3  2  1  2  3
5  4  2  1  3  4  8  4  4  0  1
0  5  8  3  1  8  4  5  6  0  5
0  5  3  3  0  4  1  3  9  2  2
6  8  3  6  9  9  4  3  0  3  5
7  7  2  9  2  3  6  7  8  4  2
8  9  4  6  1  4  5  3  1  9  4
6  9  5  4  6  7  4  5  6  5  9
3  0  8  2  5  8  3  4  5  5  3
2  7  7  1  0  1  0  1  3  5  4
0  2  7  5  3  2  5  3  4  6  8
```

NUMBER SEARCH 5

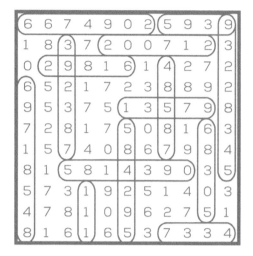

```
6  6  7  4  9  0  2  5  9  3  9
1  8  3  7  2  0  0  7  1  2  3
0  2  9  8  1  6  1  4  2  7  2
6  5  2  1  7  2  3  8  8  9  2
9  5  3  7  5  1  3  5  7  9  8
7  2  8  1  7  5  0  8  1  6  3
1  5  7  4  0  8  6  7  9  8  4
8  1  5  8  1  4  3  9  0  3  5
5  7  3  1  9  2  5  1  4  0  3
4  7  8  1  0  9  6  2  7  5  1
8  1  6  1  6  5  3  7  3  3  4
```

NUMBER SEARCH 4

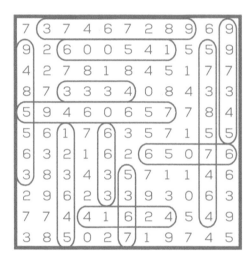

```
7  3  7  4  6  7  2  8  9  6  9
9  2  6  0  0  5  4  1  5  5  9
4  2  7  8  1  8  4  5  1  7  7
8  7  3  3  3  4  0  8  4  3  3
5  9  4  6  0  6  5  7  7  8  4
5  6  1  7  6  3  5  7  1  5  5
6  3  2  1  6  2  6  5  0  7  6
3  8  3  4  3  5  7  1  1  4  6
2  9  6  2  3  3  9  3  0  6  3
7  7  4  4  1  6  2  4  5  4  9
3  8  5  0  2  7  1  9  7  4  5
```

Number Fill-Ins

NUMBER FILL-IN 1

3	2	1	■	2	3	4	9
8	9	0	■	1	2	4	3
5	4	0	4	7	■	6	7
■	■	3	9	■	6	5	9
9	5	4	■	5	7	■	■
7	7	■	5	4	8	9	7
5	8	2	3	■	8	2	3
2	3	4	5	■	5	5	4

NUMBER FILL-IN 3

4	2	5	■	8	6	5	3
7	5	4	■	4	1	8	3
6	3	■	1	3	0	■	■
3	5	8	9	■	3	4	7
4	6	8	■	1	6	5	0
■	■	5	7	3	■	1	2
9	6	7	8	■	3	4	0
1	4	5	1	■	6	7	8

NUMBER FILL-IN 2

3	5	6	■	7	4	4	5
5	7	7	■	1	0	7	8
3	1	6	■	3	7	4	8
■	1	2	3	4	■	■	■
■	■	■	7	6	8	9	■
2	4	3	5	■	4	9	6
4	5	7	8	■	5	0	5
8	5	6	2	■	7	5	4

NUMBER FILL-IN 4

3	6	5	■	7	8	5	■
1	2	4	■	3	4	6	7
2	0	4	7	5	■	4	6
■	■	3	4	■	5	9	2
8	7	4	■	2	3	■	■
8	5	■	6	9	8	2	8
4	3	2	0	■	1	9	2
■	5	4	8	■	3	4	5

NUMBER FILL-IN 5

3	4			6	7	2	8
5	6		4	5	7	9	2
5	4	1	0	2	4		
5	6	7		2	0	2	
	2	1	5		6	4	6
		4	3	5	5	1	4
4	3	5	7	0		2	3
2	5	0	7			1	5

CHALLENGE LEVEL 2

Sudokus

SUDOKU 6

5	7	9	6	2	8	4	1	3
3	1	2	7	9	4	8	5	6
6	4	8	5	3	1	9	7	2
9	8	6	1	4	5	2	3	7
4	2	5	9	7	3	1	6	8
1	3	7	2	8	6	5	9	4
2	6	4	3	5	9	7	8	1
8	5	1	4	6	7	3	2	9
7	9	3	8	1	2	6	4	5

SUDOKU 8

3	5	8	4	9	7	6	2	1
7	4	6	2	3	1	5	9	8
2	1	9	8	6	5	4	3	7
8	7	3	1	4	6	9	5	2
4	6	5	9	2	8	7	1	3
1	9	2	7	5	3	8	4	6
6	2	1	5	7	9	3	8	4
5	3	4	6	8	2	1	7	9
9	8	7	3	1	4	2	6	5

SUDOKU 7

5	2	7	4	9	3	6	1	8
6	3	9	8	1	5	4	2	7
1	8	4	7	6	2	3	9	5
3	1	8	2	4	9	7	5	6
9	4	6	5	7	8	1	3	2
2	7	5	6	3	1	9	8	4
7	5	3	9	8	6	2	4	1
4	9	2	1	5	7	8	6	3
8	6	1	3	2	4	5	7	9

SUDOKU 9

6	1	3	9	7	5	2	8	4
9	8	2	1	3	4	7	6	5
4	5	7	8	2	6	3	9	1
2	4	8	7	5	1	9	3	6
7	6	1	3	4	9	5	2	8
3	9	5	6	8	2	1	4	7
1	2	4	5	9	8	6	7	3
8	7	6	2	1	3	4	5	9
5	3	9	4	6	7	8	1	2

SUDOKU 10

1	7	9	5	6	8	2	3	4
2	6	8	7	3	4	1	5	9
5	4	3	1	2	9	8	7	6
7	3	6	9	8	2	4	1	5
9	5	2	4	1	6	3	8	7
4	8	1	3	5	7	9	6	2
6	9	5	8	4	1	7	2	3
3	1	4	2	7	5	6	9	8
8	2	7	6	9	3	5	4	1

Number Searches

NUMBER SEARCH 6

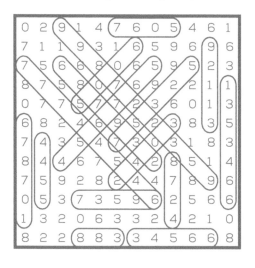

NUMBER SEARCH 7

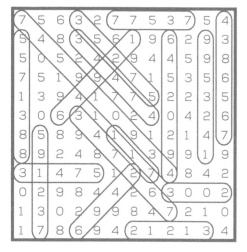

NUMBER SEARCH 8

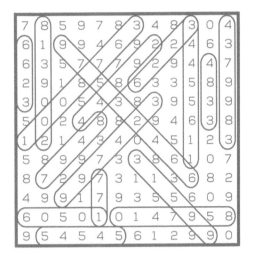

NUMBER SEARCH 10

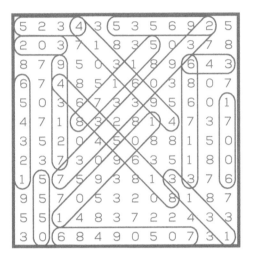

NUMBER SEARCH 9

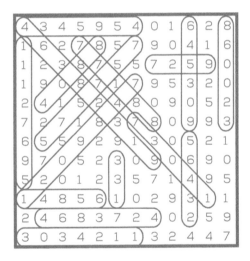

Number Fill-Ins

NUMBER FILL-IN 6

3	9	7		4	5	3		7	6	5
1	0	1		9	1	8		4	4	5
3	1	6	4	8	6	9		8	7	6
			4	8	3	7	6	2	7	5
4	5	3	9	0	0		4	4		
6	5	4	9				3	2	5	6
	3	2		9	4	8	5	7	0	
2	4	5	9	6	9	7	4			
3	8	6		2	5	9	1	2	1	6
4	1	0		5	6	4		2	2	3
3	3	5		8	6	5		7	7	7

NUMBER FILL-IN 8

5	4	9	7	1		3	4	4	3	
6	1	9	7	6		3	0	3	3	4
9	4	8		2	3	1	8	1	4	0
5	2	5	4		9	8	6			
		2	7	1		1	9	3	4	
4	6	7	7	4		3	8	4	7	5
4	1	0	5		4	9	6			
		1	7	7		7	5	4	3	
5	6	7	8	4	3	4		9	3	4
4	2	3	7	8		2	5	6	6	7
	7	1	2	0		3	5	0	6	5

NUMBER FILL-IN 7

1	4	5		7	4	5		7	9	2
2	3	2		4	1	6		7	5	4
3	1	1	5	0		3	5	2	1	0
	9	9	4	5			9	7	8	7
1	9	0	3	4	4	6	7			
3	7	0	7	3		8	4	5	7	8
	4	8	5	7	3	0	3	4		
9	2	8	1		3	2	9	1		
6	7	5	4	9		5	4	6	3	1
5	4	8		6	1	1		6	8	0
4	3	2		7	8	9		8	6	1

NUMBER FILL-IN 9

2	3	7		5	9	7		6	4	1
8	0	6		2	3	8		5	5	4
6	5	4	2	8	1	1		9	2	3
		4	8	6	5	3	1			
7	8	7	3	4		2	3	9	1	1
3	5	2						3	6	5
1	7	8	5	4		8	7	3	3	4
	5	0	7	5	4	2				
2	4	4		7	2	0	3	8	7	5
2	6	3		1	0	0		2	5	6
3	4	2		2	7	6		7	3	3

NUMBER FILL-IN 10

2	4		7	4	5		9	1	2	3
2	0	9	8	3	6		2	3	1	1
8	6	3	5	0	8		2	3	7	5
2	3	4		5	7	4	5	6	0	2
1	3	6	8		8	5	3			
2	5	7	3	9		8	4	5	3	9
		8	0	9		2	1	6	5	
7	6	3	4	8	9	3		3	0	7
7	5	3	1		2	1	3	8	5	2
5	3	7	8		8	1	2	6	3	5
6	4	3	8		3	0	9		4	4

CHALLENGE LEVEL 3

Sudokus

SUDOKU 11

5	8	7	3	6	4	2	9	1
1	4	6	9	8	2	5	3	7
9	2	3	7	5	1	8	4	6
2	3	9	4	7	8	1	6	5
4	5	8	1	3	6	7	2	9
6	7	1	5	2	9	4	8	3
7	6	5	2	4	3	9	1	8
3	9	4	8	1	7	6	5	2
8	1	2	6	9	5	3	7	4

SUDOKU 13

8	3	4	5	6	9	7	1	2
9	6	7	3	1	2	4	5	8
5	1	2	8	4	7	3	9	6
7	9	8	6	2	5	1	3	4
6	4	1	9	7	3	8	2	5
2	5	3	1	8	4	6	7	9
1	2	9	4	3	6	5	8	7
3	7	6	2	5	8	9	4	1
4	8	5	7	9	1	2	6	3

SUDOKU 12

7	9	5	1	4	8	3	2	6
3	4	6	7	2	9	1	8	5
1	8	2	5	3	6	4	7	9
6	3	7	2	8	4	5	9	1
8	2	9	3	1	5	6	4	7
5	1	4	6	9	7	8	3	2
4	7	1	8	5	2	9	6	3
2	5	8	9	6	3	7	1	4
9	6	3	4	7	1	2	5	8

SUDOKU 14

4	8	5	9	2	1	3	6	7
6	3	9	7	5	8	1	2	4
2	1	7	4	6	3	8	9	5
1	4	3	2	7	5	9	8	6
5	2	8	3	9	6	7	4	1
7	9	6	8	1	4	5	3	2
3	6	4	5	8	7	2	1	9
8	5	2	1	4	9	6	7	3
9	7	1	6	3	2	4	5	8

SUDOKU 15

7	3	2	4	8	6	5	1	9
6	5	4	3	1	9	2	7	8
8	9	1	2	5	7	6	3	4
3	2	7	5	9	4	1	8	6
5	4	8	6	7	1	3	9	2
9	1	6	8	3	2	7	4	5
4	7	5	9	2	3	8	6	1
2	6	3	1	4	8	9	5	7
1	8	9	7	6	5	4	2	3

Number Searches

NUMBER SEARCH 11

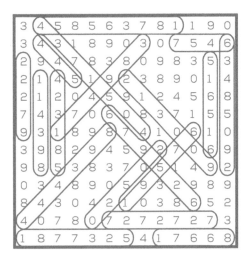

NUMBER SEARCH 12

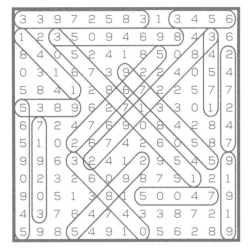

NUMBER SEARCH 13

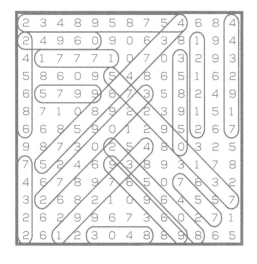

NUMBER SEARCH 15

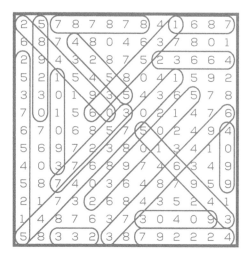

NUMBER SEARCH 14

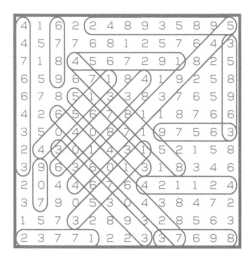

Number Fill-Ins

NUMBER FILL-IN 11

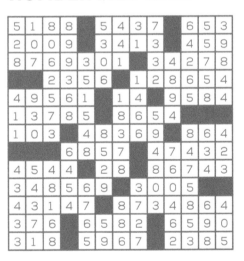

```
    3 7 4     2 7 6     3 2 1
2 0 3 8     1 9 4     6 2 8 7
5 4 9 3 7 8 5 6     4 8 5 7
1 0 9 3 8     3 8 3 4 0 2 5
        2 1 3       5 9 5
4 5 2 9 4 5 8 5 8     4 1 1
6 3 2 8     6 9 8     3 2 1 0
8 3 3     4 5 2 4 9 5 6 6 0
      9 5 6       2 8 4
5 3 2 1 1 5 6     2 1 5 4 8
8 7 6 6     7 5 4 3 1 7 6 7
1 2 9 0     4 3 2     8 7 7 2
    3 4 5     2 3 8     5 4 6
```

NUMBER FILL-IN 13

```
7 5 9 6 8     3 4 1     6 9 8
3 0 1 3 5     4 2 0     4 3 2
2 4 1 6 9     8 3 7     4 5 0
1 1 4     1 6 8     5 4 8 9
      3 9 4     5 5 6 6
9 3 8 2 0     3 5 6 4 3 1 2
4 9 5 6     4 5 6     8 4 7 4
3 5 7 5 4 8 3     1 2 3 8 5
      5 5 2 8     9 5 8
4 4 8 3       5 8 1     3 4 2
7 9 4     3 5 6     8 6 4 3 6
1 0 0     3 4 5     7 5 4 3 6
4 9 0     8 7 5     6 8 7 5 3
```

NUMBER FILL-IN 12

```
5 1 8 8     5 4 3 7     6 5 3
2 0 0 9     3 4 1 3     4 5 9
8 7 6 9 3 0 1     3 4 2 7 8
      2 3 5 6     1 2 8 6 5 4
4 9 5 6 1     1 4     9 5 8 4
1 3 7 8 5     8 6 5 4
1 0 3     4 8 3 6 9     8 6 4
      6 8 5 7     4 7 4 3 2
4 5 4 4     2 8     8 6 7 4 3
3 4 8 5 6 9     3 0 0 5
4 3 1 4 7     8 7 3 4 8 6 4
3 7 6     6 5 8 2     6 5 9 0
3 1 8     5 9 6 7     2 3 8 5
```

NUMBER FILL-IN 14

```
3 9 4 6 9     2 1 6     5 6 4
2 4 8 3 1     3 2 7     5 6 8
2 4 5 8 1     6 0 8     4 6 3
5 6 1     5 9 7 8     7 8 2 3
      2 9 5 6 8 7 3
9 3 7 4 4 5     3 8 7 2 4 9
3 1 2 5       8 3 7 4
9 0 3 7 8 4     3 2 5 7 5 4
      4 8 5 6 7 0 2
5 9 6 3     9 0 8 6     2 3 6
4 4 6     7 8 5     2 2 6 7 8
1 2 3     5 5 6     7 4 2 4 7
9 0 7     3 4 6     2 6 4 6 8
```

NUMBER FILL-IN 15

3	5	5	8	■	2	4	9	■	4	3	2	8
2	4	7	2	■	5	0	8	■	7	2	7	6
4	8	2	5	8	5	4	4	■	2	3	5	1
■	■	■	1	2	9	■	4	8	2	1	0
1	2	1	4	8	■	3	2	9	8	■	■	■
3	2	5	7	■	1	0	9	4	7	4	7
2	6	8	9	2	3	■	9	6	1	3	4	1
8	0	7	6	4	5	3	■	2	3	4	6
■	■	2	1	2	6	■	1	5	7	8	9
3	9	5	1	6	■	4	1	9	■	■	■
6	8	3	4	■	4	7	4	5	2	4	5	8
5	0	0	3	■	2	9	5	■	5	1	9	8
2	3	4	7	■	1	6	4	■	4	8	9	4

RESOURCES

Check out these resources for more ideas on fun, helpful, and engaging activities:

Of Course!: The Greatest Collection of Riddles & Brain Teasers for Expanding Your Mind by Zack Guido is a collection of riddles, puzzles, and brain teasers to challenge your mind and introduce you to new ways of thinking.

Large Print Coloring Book: Easy Patterns for Adults by Dylanna Press features pages of line drawings that offer opportunity for creative coloring while flexing your fine motor skills.

Moonwalking with Einstein: The Art and Science of Remembering Everything by Joshua Foer follows a man's journey to remember everything, and is packed with science and techniques to improve memory.

Bouncing Back: Skills for Adaptation to Injury, Aging, Illness, and Pain by Richard Wanlass, PhD, is an excellent user-friendly guide to helpful strategies and information related to its titled topic.

Radiolab with Jad Abumrad and Robert Krulwich (WNYC Studios) is a podcast that entertains on topics of everyday interest with lighthearted commentary and lots of factual details.

The Mindful Awareness Research Center at University of California, Los Angeles (UCLAHealth.org/marc/) is a rich resource for useful webinars, podcasts, guided meditations, and more on the theory and practice of mindful awareness.

REFERENCES

Coles-Brennan, C., A. Sulley, and G. Young. "Management of Digital Eye Strain." *Clinical and Experimental Optometry* 102(1) (2019): 18–29.

Firth, J., B. Stubbs, D. Vancampfort, F. Schuch, J. Lagopoulos, S. Rosenbaum, and P. B. Ward. "Effect of Aerobic Exercise on Hippocampal Volume in Humans: A Systematic Review and Meta-analysis." *Neuroimage* 166 (2018): 230–38.

Goble, D. J., J. P. Coxon, N. Wenderoth, A. Van Impe, and S. P. Swinnen. "Proprioceptive Sensibility in the Elderly: Degeneration, Functional Consequences and Plastic-Adaptive Processes." *Neuroscience & Biobehavioral Reviews* 33(3) (2009): 271–78.

Hall, C. B., R. B. Lipton, M. Sliwinski, M. J. Katz, C. A. Derby, and J. Verghese. "Cognitive Activities Delay Onset of Memory Decline in Persons Who Develop Dementia." *Neurology* 73(5) (2009): 356–61.

Hoang, T. D., J. Reis, N. Zhu, D. R. Jacobs, L. J. Launer, R. A. Whitmer, S. Sidney, and K. Yaffe. "Effect of Early Adult Patterns of Physical Activity and Television Viewing on Midlife Cognitive Function." *JAMA Psychiatry* 73(1) (2016): 73–79.

Humes, L. E., and L. A. Young. "Sensory-Cognitive Interactions in Older Adults." *Ear and Hearing* 37(Suppl 1) (2016): 52S–61S.

Krueger, K. R., R. S. Wilson, J. M. Kamenetsky, L. L. Barnes, J. L. Bienias, and D. A. Bennett. "Social Engagement and Cognitive Function in Old Age." *Experimental Aging Research* 35(1) (2009): 45–60.

Lo, J. C., D. J. Dijk, and J. A. Groeger. "Comparing the Effects of Nocturnal Sleep and Daytime Napping on Declarative Memory Consolidation." *PLoS One* 9(9) (2014): e108100.

Lu, J. G., M. Akinola, and M. F. Mason. "'Switching On' Creativity: Task Switching Can Increase Creativity by Reducing Cognitive Fixation." *Organizational Behavior and Human Decision Processes* 139 (2017): 63–75.

McEvoy, C. T., H. Guyer, K. M. Langa, and K. Yaffe. "Neuroprotective Diets Are Associated with Better Cognitive Function: The Health and Retirement Study." *Journal of the American Geriatrics Society* 65(8) (2017): 1857–62.

Sacks, O. *Musicophilia: Tales of Music and the Brain*. New York: Vintage Books, 2007.

Schultz, S. A., J. Larson, J. Oh, R. Koscik, M. N. Dowling, C. L. Gallagher, C. M. Carlsson, et al. "Participation in Cognitively-Stimulating Activities Is Associated with Brain Structure and Cognitive Function in Preclinical Alzheimer's Disease." *Brain Imaging and Behavior* 9(4) (2015): 729–36.

Stradley, L. "History of Cookies." *What's Cooking America*. July 12, 2020. WhatsCookingAmerica.net/History/CookieHistory.htm.

Toepfer, S. M., K. Cichy, and P. Peters. "Letters of Gratitude: Further Evidence for Author Benefits." *Journal of Happiness Studies* 13(1) (2012): 187–201.

Wijndaele, K., S. Brage, H. Besson, K. T. Khaw, S. J. Sharp, R. Luben, N. J. Wareham, and U. Ekelund. "Television Viewing Time Independently Predicts All-Cause and Cardiovascular Mortality: The EPIC Norfolk Study." *International Journal of Epidemiology* 40(1) (2011): 150–59.

INDEX

ACKNOWLEDGMENTS

What a fun project this has been. I looked forward to working on this book each time I set out to do so, which is largely in response to the individuals involved in this project. From my first conversation with Wesley Chiu at Callisto Media, to ongoing coordination with my editors Lori Tenny and Laurie White, I felt inspired and encouraged. I'd like to thank Phil Fraas for his dedication to making the puzzles challenging and accessible through his excellent communication and puzzle-making skill. I truly had a great team.

I'd also like to thank those who have filled my mind with experiences in clinical and academic work. A big thank-you to Dr. Erik Lande for his ongoing mentorship across the years, and to Dr. Richard Wanlass; both mentors modeled for me that writing a book is an enjoyable feat that can be rewarding to its author and readers.

A warm thank-you to my family and friends who served as constructive critics for the numerous and varied activity ideas I put on the drawing board. *Xiexie* to Shera and *merci* to Anahita for your linguistic talents. Thank you, Jon, for keeping me company on those long writing days. I'm thankful to have a mom with an editing background and a thirst for wisdom, a dad willing to test-drive whatever activity I threw at him, and a brother with whom I've shared decades of creative endeavors.

ABOUT THE AUTHOR

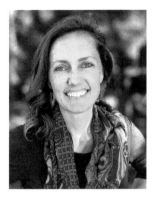

Alexis Olson, PhD, specializes in neuropsychological evaluations and therapy for individuals affected by brain injury, chronic pain/illness, and caregiving.

Fueled by a desire to increase patient access to information and opportunities for brain wellness, she compiled this book using many of the tips and techniques she implements in her work with patients and their loved ones.

Dr. Olson regularly provides cognitive training, involving learning and practicing compensatory cognitive strategies in everyday life situations. Her background includes a PhD in clinical psychology from the University of California, Santa Barbara, and postdoctoral training at UC Davis Medical Center Physical Medicine and Rehabilitation Department, as well as at Advanced Neurobehavioral Health in coordination with University of California, San Diego.

Dr. Olson is a published researcher in the field of rehabilitation psychology. She is a national presenter and active researcher on the topic of brain function and adult protective services. She is currently a neuropsychologist in the San Diego area, where she wrote most of this book while breathing in the salty air on Mission Bay. Find out more about Dr. Alexis Olson at DoctorOlson.com.

ABOUT THE PUZZLE AUTHOR

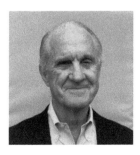

Phil Fraas is a longtime constructor of crossword puzzles. He started in the early 1980s when he had several of his first efforts published in the *New York Times*. He now oversees and constructs puzzles for a free crossword, sudoku, and word search puzzle website—YourPuzzleSource.com.

CPSIA information can be obtained
at www.ICGtesting.com
Printed in the USA
LVHW021208150321
681247LV00001B/1

9 781647 397258